The Divine SelfCare Strategy

The Divine SelfQare Strategy

A Wellness Guide to Total Body Alignment

By Sheila Brown, JD

Published By Lighthouse Consulting, LLC

Bethesda, Maryland

Copyright © 2022

Disclaimer

Sheila Brown, JD Copyright © 2022 – All Rights Reserved

Copyright © Sheila Brown, JD 2022

No part of this book may be reproduced, stored, or transmitted in any form or by any means, including mechanical or electronic, without prior written permission from the author.

While the author has made every effort to ensure that the ideas, statistics, and information presented in this book are accurate to the best of her abilities, any implications direct, derived, or perceived, should only be used by the reader's discretion. The author cannot be held responsible for any personal or commercial damage arising from communication, application, or misinterpretation of the information presented herein.

All Rights Reserved
Library of Congress Control Number: 2022910130
ISBN 9798218000271
Created in the United States of America
Lighthouse Consulting LLC
DBA/Queendom Qare LLC
Attn: Sheila Brown, JD
4701 Sangamore Road Suite 100N #2007
Bethesda, Maryland 20816
Email info@queendomqare.com
Phone (202) 952-6123
Printed in the United States of America
First Edition

For you, mom,

A Note from the Author

When I received my results from the bar exam in December of 2009, I was so excited because I thought my career as an estate-planning attorney would kick off in Atlanta, GA. I had done the impossible. I graduated from Texas Southern University, Thurgood Marshall School of law school in the top 25% of my class as a single mother in an unfamiliar state with very few resources other than hope, effective management skills, and a sheer will to succeed. When I got to Atlanta, I was pushed into an unfamiliar area of work for me called corporate strategic planning. I didn't choose it, but it seemed to have chosen me, and I am so glad it did. The work and the painful learning experiences associated with it catapulted my natural intuition into a more deliberate framework providing a new way of thinking and approaching the world and even my personal problems.

Had I had such a systemic approach to analyzing the issues that arose in my life at 18, I am not sure how things may have turned out for me. But I trust that my path in life was guided by the divine hand of the Most High, and every lesson in it was meant for good. One of the greatest goods was writing this book. There was a saying that I learned in my youth. It was, **"The enemy has a plan. The Most High has a plan. But thankfully, the Most High is the best of planners."**

The book you are holding in your hand is forged from the wisdom of a woman who has lived four lifetimes in just 44 years. Looking back through time, as I did over the course of writing the chapters of this book, also forced me to examine some important milestones in my life and analyze the people who showed up in the chapters of my four crucial decades to instill a lesson that would form the pages of this timeless wisdom called the *Divine SelfQare Strategy: A Wellness Guide To Total Body Alignment*. This is such an imperfect title but in a good way. It certainly does meet its goal of defining true wellness and laying the uncommon roadmap that leads to what is called *Total Body Alignment* in women. But what the title falls short of doing is describing the incredible journey you are about to take with me as a reader.

You might not know it, but this book is written towards the future; for people I haven't met yet, but who I hope with all fervor and faith will be as real one day as you and I are now. It is written for my future grandchildren, and generations of offspring that I pray are to come from them so that they will know me as their matriarch and so that they will deeply know themselves. When I was a little girl, I had a great-grandmother who loved me deeply. She loved me so much that she would get up at 5 am every morning and bathe me. I know that might not seem like evidence for a claim of love, but it is. Time was my great-grandmother's love language, and spending time with the precious great-granddaughter she loved as an infant meant everything to her. She prayed over me and wished nothing but the best life for me with every breath she took. Then there was my grandmother, Betty, the great connector.

I didn't realize it at the time of my youth, but every story she told over and over again was to keep me connected to something beyond me and time. She kept telling me these stories, some of which you will hear about later. Stories that conveyed imagery of resilient women, brilliant women with special gifts of healing from nature's basic resources, filled my young imagination. As my grandmother orated these stories, I didn't know how powerful they were or how critical they would become over the next few decades of my life, but they were, and time proves it. This book also proves it.

Another reason why this book title falls short of the power of its contents is that it doesn't *fully* convey to you as a prospective reader all about the mysteries shown to me from my studies of the texts, poems, speeches, biographies, reference books, articles, and songs of our ancestors. Such wonderful revelations I uncovered that just have to be read to be believed and understood for yourself. So, there is a whole chapter dedicated to laying an ancient foundation for the work we are to do for our own healing and self-care as women.

This foundation is so profound that I must confess this was the hardest chapter to write. It was also the most compelling chapter for me to write, and when it was done, I was convinced that the *Divine SelfQare Strategy* was going to succeed at the goal of opening the minds of young people to their rich heritage and medicinal legacy as custodians of the earth and its vast resources gifted to us by the Most High. In this chapter, you will be surprised to hear how our ancestors chose to engage with '**A.F.E.W.**' tools, an acronym for the four elements, ***air, fire, earth,*** and ***water***, to achieve freedom and conquer health issues. Expect to be immersed in an interconnected theme of power, science, and wisdom through the works of the honorable Frederick Douglas, Reverend Dr. Martin Luther King, Jr., Queen Mother Harriet Tubman, and Queen Mother Harriet Jacobs, among others.

This lays the foundation through our collective ancestors that, once revealed, will make so much sense in the great scheme of things called history and survival in the face of brutal oppression from slavery, Jim Crow, and medical apartheid as Harriet Washington, the great author of the book by the same title put it. But why was it necessary to go there with these ancestors for a book purportedly about Total Body Alignment? You'll understand why in chapters four and five when the most comprehensive discussion of the ancestral wisdom of the four natural resources is broken down and how when coupled with the most important spiritual element called Divine Intention come into play. This early work is important because it gives meaning to everything recommended to support women's bodily wellness, mental and spiritual health, and overall relationships that contribute to well-being. Choices have to be made young. And the sooner our youth know this information, the better their chances are of thriving in the world and not merely surviving it - oftentimes so full of regrets later in life.

The world was full of wonders and dangers when I was young; today, it is even more so. So, the relationship between *Divine SelfQare* and freedom takes on another dimension. The Total Body Alignment system teaches women that they need to see *and* have vision, hear *and* listen, and talk *and* speak with intention. The eyes, ears, mouth, and nose become viewed as vital resources connected to our spiritual sense of sight, speech, and listening skills. Therefore, it may not be popular, but it is necessary to state that one should and must refrain from beauty standards obstructing these sensory organs. Total Body Alignment is not a momentary accomplishment; it is something we strive toward each day of our lives as we set out to fulfill our divine purpose.

I hope you enjoy reading this book. It was written from the perspective of me as an aging grandmother, one who may or may not be alive in the flesh when the intended audience, my beautiful *grands* and *great-great grands* will prayerfully exist. It was hard to imagine what the world would look like 200 years from now, but I envisioned my descendants, my precious grandchildren, still closely aligned to the divine principles that make us the children of the Most High. In a way, all children, whether yours or mine, are connected to me and are the intended audiences of this book as well. But imagining that I was writing for a narrower audience, knowing that I intended for the world to read it, enabled me to reveal myself more. I was able to become vulnerable and transparent. For anyone who knows me personally, the understanding of why this was such an accomplishment for me will become evident.

I hope that no matter who holds this book, it will be a reminder and a blessing of how simple yet satisfying life and health can be when we strive to live in harmony with the bounty of nature as given to us for stewardship by the Creator of all life on earth and in heaven.

Finally, I would like to acknowledge the love and support I received from family, friends, well-wishers, and of course, the many professionals whose gift of editing, proofing, designing, video creation, and marketing - coupled with a healthy dose of patience - made all of this divine work that I can now present to the world possible. Thank you!

Peace and blessings. Enjoy this special journey with me as you turn the page.

Sheila Brown, JD
Washington, DC
May 8, 2022

CONTENTS

Chapter 1   1
Introduction   2
Chapter 2   11
Grandmother Betty   12
  Salted Pork Fat & Copper Pennies   13
  Rotten Apples & Witch Hazel   15
  Spirits of Turpentine   16
  Grandmother Rebecca Did Not Play Games   17
  Grandmother Betty and the Neighbor   19
  A Grandbaby's Half Dollar Navel   22
Chapter 3   25
Voice of the Ancestors   26
  Ancestral Perspectives on the Four Elements   27
    Frederick Douglas Speaks   29
    Reverend Dr. Martin Luther King Speaks   33
  Trans-physics in Practice | Healing Ways and Freedom   38
    Queen Mother Harriet Tubman Speaks   39
    Queen Mother Harriet Jacobs Speaks   49
  The Story Of Sally Brown   55
  The Story of Gus Smith   58
  A Rivalry with Western Medicine   61
  The Honorable Marcus Garvey Speaks   65
Chapter 4   67
Air | Fire | Earth | Water   68
  Trans-physics Defined   70
  A.F.E.W. | Qualities & Characteristics   75
    Air   77
    Fire   79
    Earth   81
    Water   83
Chapter 5   87
Fifth Element | Divine Intention   88
  Clean Face | Pure Heart   90
  Clean Face | Impure Heart   93
  Unclean Face | Pure Heart   96

Unclean Face | Impure Heart	97
Divine Intention | Wicked Intention	104
Face	104
Heart	109
Clean | Unclean	112
Pure | Impure	114

Chapter 6 — 119

Sacred Wellness	120
Head | Womb | Feet	120
African Origins of Divine SelfQare | The Awakening	125
Quest for Truth | Journey in the Aisles	130
Queen Of Thousands | Yeshimebet Speaks	135

Chapter 7 — 141

Denkenesh	142

Chapter 8 — 149

Total Body Alignment	150
The Art Of Total Body Alignment| Grounded | Centered | Elevated	154
Denkenesh| Woman Of Divine Imagination	157
Denkenesh | Cycle of Divine Womanhood	159
Denkenesh | Exemplar of Divine Relationships	163
Denkenesh | Pillars of Divine Health	166
A Beautiful & Wonderful Sacred Temple	172
A Guide To The Body As A Sacred Temple	175
Crown | Head	176
Throne | Womb	192
Pedestal | Feet	197
Treasures Of Sacred Knowledge	200
Create Your Personal Divine SelfQare Environment	206

Chapter 9 — 213

Divine SelfQare Overview	214
The Sacred Temple	218
The Head As A Sacred Crown	218
The Womb As A Royal Throne	218
The Feet As A Grand Pedestal	219
Divine SelfQare Routine | Schedule	220
Divine SelfQare Methods	221
Cleanse The Crown | Achieve Elevation	221

Eye Qleanse	221
Ear Qleanse	224
Oral Qleanse	226
Nasal & Upper Respiratory Qleanse | Facial Detox	228
Cleanse The Throne | Achieve Centering	230
Welcome Womb Wellness	230
The Top 5 Challenges to Being Centered In Vaginal Wellness	231
Womb Qleanse Vaginal Steaming As An At-Home Therapeutic Treatment	233
The Art of Jeweling	235
Exercise 1	239
Exercise 2	241
Exercise 3	243
Exercise 4	245
Exercise 5	247
Cleanse The Pedestal | Achieve Grounding	250
Focus On Feet	250
Foot Qleanse	250
The Tools Of Wellness Through Divine SelfQare	253
Qrown Qare	255
Eye Masq	255
Oral Qare Cleansers	256
Ear Qones or Ear Qandles	257
Qrown Qare Steam Station	258
Throne Qare	260
Throne Qare Steam Station	260
Plush Pillow	261
Herbal Blends	262
Throne Jewels	263
Steam Gown	264
Pedestal Qare	265
Foot Basin	265
Foot Soak Salts	266
Immerse Yourself In Wellness	267
Epilogue	269
Divine Closure	270
Glossary	273

> "If there's a book you want to read,
> but it hasn't been written yet,
> then you must write it."
> Toni Morrison

Chapter 1

Introduction

My Dear Grandchildren,

I've loved you since before you were born.

To write this book with the hopes of you reading it one day is the driving force that has kept me determined to complete this important work after all these years. The time in which I pen down my thoughts, I am yet to be a grandmother. My faith in the Most High, coupled with my promising son, Zakur, fuels my hopes of one day becoming the grand matriarch over a thriving family full of healthy granddaughters and grandsons.

I address these carefully curated words to my future grandchildren, whom it will be the greatest pleasure to hold in my arms one day. Among all that I do not know, I somehow feel confident that my beautiful grandchildren will be proud to pass on the knowledge that I seek to share with them through this book.

Although this book is written primarily as guidance for my granddaughters, I want to equally welcome my grandsons to read it and impart this knowledge to their future wives, daughters, and perhaps any friends who may benefit from the wisdom it contains. There is nothing more than I would like than for this book to be a gift for the generations to come. Divine Health is everyone's birthright, and *Divine SelfQare* is for any woman who embraces it.

Like my grandmother before me, I want to be the beacon of our ancestral knowledge that helps the wisdom flow from one generation of strong, beautiful women to another. Therefore, I chose to write this book on *Divine SelfQare* to share with you, my beautiful daughters, what it means to be a practitioner of Divine Health.

As you bloom and come of age, I want this book to be a companion and guide to help you along the way. *A Divine SelfQare Strategy* to provide you with the knowledge of your ancestors fused with the advancements of the modern world.

I want you to grow to be strong, kind, compassionate, and, most importantly, in touch with your roots. You must remember, beautiful daughters, to find your true self, you must know who the women before you were.

*"For I am my mother's daughter,
and the drums of Africa still beat in my heart."
Mary McLeod Bethune*

It is the past that forges the future, and without it, we are empty. My daughters, the Sankofa bird, is a symbol to remind us we must remember the past as we continue to move forward. At the same time, we must plant the seed of knowledge for the generation to come after us. The bird's beautiful neck turning backward highlights the Ghanaian concept of never leaving the jewels of the past behind.

Much like the concept of the mythical bird *Sankofa*, you must go back and fetch the knowledge of your lineage to achieve the basis of optimal health and wellness.

As women of Divine Health, we have to learn how to take care of our bodies. Unfortunately, modern practices have entirely changed the way women treat themselves. Painful treatments and unnecessary procedures, only to further nip and tuck at our bodies, have become the definition of self-care and beauty.

My daughters, you must view your body as a temple. A sacred place that needs to be nourished with Divine Health and *Divine SelfQare*. Through this book, I want to convey to you that there is both a physical and spiritual basis to achieving optimal health.

I, and your great grandmothers before me, strongly believe in Divine Health as being the ultimate *SelfQare* goal.

Divine Health is a state of physical excellence, a sound mind, and spiritual balance. Its practices are not restricted to any age and can benefit anyone who accepts it as a right of way.

In all my years as a Health and Wellness practitioner, I have accumulated and put into practice the wisdom of *Divine SelfQare* and Divine Health.

Through breaking the norms of traditional self-care, I incorporated my understanding of the fundamentals of health into my work.

I would rely on the natural modalities of healing with elements that nature gifted us. With my work, I realized that maintaining and healing bodily diseases with the four primary tools found in nature is part of *Divine SelfQare* on the journey toward achieving a state of Divine Health.

The four tools I speak of are **Air, Fire, Earth**, and **Water,** or "**A.F.E.W.**" tools. We are very fortunate that the elements are abundantly available on our planet to use to our advantage.

My precious granddaughters, your perception of self-care and bodily health may be facials, hair treatments, manicures, and pedicures that result in surface beauty. While there is nothing wrong with beautification, you must understand that these practices are based on exposure to harmful chemicals that potentially lead to adverse health conditions.

The Divine SelfQare Strategy teaches you to use the natural elements to heal, maintain, beautify, and rejuvenate your body, mind, and spirit. Therefore, my daughters, I want you to wield the elements like you would wield a mighty sword and use them as a solution against disease or anything that stands in the way of you and your Divine Health.

Employing the four elements as a part of *Divine SelfQare* dates back thousands of years when the earliest people on the continent of Africa were known to exist. Healing and prevention strategies with the four elements have worked for generations before us. With the right seed of knowledge, they will work for the generations that are yet to come.

With **A.F.E.W.** tools, ancient healing modalities, and the wisdom of the Most High, I have conceived the idea for this book as a road map; hence, the title *"The Divine SelfQare Strategy."*

Women like my grandmother, great grandmother, and great-great-grandmother avoided premature death and disease with the four elements, despite lacking access to formal education, medical training, or access to the medical advancements attained during their lifetimes.

As a mother, daughter, and granddaughter myself, I know firsthand what it means to be a *Divine SelfQare Practitioner*. I can tell you that our ancestors found means of surviving when there were none.

In the early parts of the 20th Century, our ancestors were battling systemic racism and the oppression inflicted on them by the US government. Regardless of the unfavorable circumstances and limited resources, the courageous women of our family did what they had to do using their creative ingenuity and little else.

It was their inventive mind and unparalleled skill that allowed them to use natural elements such as plants to create teas, poultices, and tinctures, fused with household items like vinegar and pennies to heal diseases, wounds, and bodily ailments.

There is nothing more I would like than for my descendants to read, understand, and learn from the illustrations, stories, and memoirs of the courageous women of our family who came before you.

Their stories deserve to be told, remembered, discussed, and contemplated because that is the wise thing to do. It is upon our shoulders to impart the knowledge that our family possesses to the next generation in order to benefit society and improve the world. This is what the concept of Sankofa teaches us.

As a *Divine SelfQare* practitioner, I want to teach my granddaughters how to strategically plan a pathway to a future they desire. A future where our wisdom and Divine Health help us become strong, courageous women who can prevent illness, fight disease, and help our family and others acquire and maintain a state of Divine Health and medical freedom.

May each generation to come after me allow this book to begin your journey toward a state of Divine Health rather than end mine. While writing this book, I envision future generations of mine reading it and being blessed with the wisdom of their ancestors. Each page, each chapter, each story is a passage back to a time when our ancestors consistently did what science and academia said they couldn't—effectively diagnose, treat, cure, and prevent disease.

The wise women of our family relied on plants, herbs, and other elements found in nature as well as each other to survive through times I cannot find the right words to describe. *The Divine SelfQare Strategy* exists, as does light at the end of each tunnel because of all their wisdom, strength, and beauty. So, you see, my beloved grandchildren, you are born of the same blood, and you too can access the gift of divine health as was intended for us by the Most High, who is our guide and the creator of all things.

My precious ones, I encourage you to view this book as a living document that can help you develop and archive other modalities of natural healing. With this book, you can grow your knowledge about natural medicine, Divine Health, and *Divine SelfQare*.

Remember, true wealth is having Divine Health. True happiness is having knowledge that you can impart to the world. Divine Knowledge sets you apart and helps you do better for the generations to come. I want you to expand on it, reinterpret it, and add to it what you know. You must understand, my precious grandchildren, that it is you who will carry this book on, and what you know is equally important as what your ancestors have enabled me to pass onto you by the grace of the Most High.

There are many lessons to take away from this book and the stories it contains. One of the most important lessons, however, is for you never to forget the matriarchs and cultivators of our family's healing tradition, grandmother Betty, my great-grandmother Lena Mae, and my great-great-grandmother Rebecca. I will discuss their wisdom with you as you move ahead. I want you to know that these powerful women helped shape the fabric of our lives, and it was their perseverance and hard work that helped create the conditions that keep us going every day. Let us honor their memories. Let us continue to remember their names.

It pains me to tell you that I have no more knowledge of our paternal lineage beyond these women. There is so much information from both my paternal and maternal sides of the family that has been lost to the passage of time. The rigors of segregation, systematic racism, and slavery imposed on our family led to an incomparable loss of knowledge and wisdom.

This loss is what drives me to write this book so that no other generation of our family has to ever live to grow up without the wisdom of its ancestors. My daughters, you are my descendants, and I pray that you will become women who embrace natural beauty, health, and radical self-reliance. I pray for you to have the strength and wisdom to prevent and cure disease and, when necessary, use natural treatments on your own bodies to heal, like the strong, resourceful women you have the potential to become.

Even as someone who is yet to be a grandmother, I am already proud of the women who I hope and pray you will one day become. That you will be women who dare to stay true to the values of divine womanhood, the sacred and precious daughters of the Most High. This book is my call to you to practice *Divine SelfQare,* live graciously in wellness, and prosper in the fullness of Divine Health.

I want you, my sacred granddaughters, to live to the fullest and express divine creativity in every way you choose. I hope you will subscribe to simplicity and study the modalities of natural healing along with the 19 principles of Divine Health using this book as your guide.

Let the *Divine SelfQare Strategy* take precedence when it comes to the maintenance of health. Use it to support the fulfillment of your life's divine purpose. I have written this book for you as a roadmap through which you can navigate sound principles about *Divine SelfQare* and good health. Sacred daughters, you must know that you are not alone in this world, and the challenges you face are not only yours.

With all that I have been able to retain in my mind from the wisdom of our matriarchs, I have also attempted to articulate this book in the best manner possible to help you in the future despite not knowing what that future may be.

I have something unique to offer you through this book because, having lived an extraordinary life thus far, I have overcome several challenges that may, at some point, arise in your lives too. In those moments, I want you to know that each of you possesses the wisdom, fortitude, and spiritual insights of your foremothers. This will give you the strength to pull from any difficult situation that you may be in.

As you read on, you will understand that this book holds powerful secrets. It contains all of the ancient wisdom and inherited therapeutic techniques bestowed upon me directly through tradition, divine inspiration, or my own studies.

These women, whose therapeutic practices I have studied, emerge from African ancestry and heritage. Each of these women has something unique and powerful to share about health, the body, and healing it because of what they have been through. As descendants of those resourceful formerly enslaved women, mothers, sisters, and midwives who have SURVIVED unspeakable experiences, their wisdom is the strength that graces the pages of this book.

Chapter 2

Grandmother Betty

As precious daughters of the future, you should be aware that the book you are holding in your hand is forged, in part, from the knowledge of your ancestors: paternal Great-great-grandmother Rebecca, Great-grandmother Lena Mae, Grandmother Betty, and I.

There came the point where we nearly lost everything – our ancestral lineage, genetic heritage, ancient culture, language, and traditions. Most importantly, the profound knowledge of sacred and effective healing. The unfairness of our history prevents us from calling on the names of our ancestors who precede Great-great-grandmother Rebecca on my father's side.

Similarly, I possess very little knowledge of our maternal ancestry. I never met anyone beyond my mother's mother, Mary Parker, the grandmother, who helped to raise me till the age of five. Yet, it is always important to acknowledge that they existed in spirit and truth. They exist today in our very DNA because we exist. They live on through our inherited memories and genetics.

Thankfully, some of this legacy was preserved to serve a greater divine purpose. This legacy exists in forgotten manuscripts, the diaries of plantation wives, and even books tucked away in the hidden rooms of obscure libraries. Although it is difficult to seek them out, you must remember the concept of the Sankofa: to go back and get it.

When the time comes for you to read this book, I want you to take the time to first bask in it, knowing that it is filled with the love of every matriarch who came before me. This love is expressed through some of the thoughts, sayings, and Divine Intentions that they had for you. Memories of their sound health practices and behaviors preserved here are meant to remind you to stimulate your own bodily, mental, and physical well-being.

If you pay attention, you will realize how the wisdom of our ancestors is part of our DNA. It surfaces with every move you make, with every thought you have about health and your survival. Sometimes, we don't need textbooks to make us realize the Divine Creativity that rests within us. That, my beautiful daughters, is what we call intuition. That gut feeling or intuition is also referred to as the first voice. It is actually the voice of the Most High, guiding our path in the most beautiful ways.

Today, I am ecstatic to share what Grandmother Betty passed down to me. Her stories, techniques, and beautiful naturopathic ways of utilizing minerals, essential oils, plants, and even natural food substances for healing.

Salted Pork Fat & Copper Pennies

When Grandmother Betty was a child, she aspired to be a famous singer and dancer. As she grew older, her voice and physique were a testament to the fact that she was meant for it.

Unfortunately, while playing with other kids from her community, Grandmother Betty stumbled on top of a large, rusty nail protruding from the ground that pierced right through her tennis shoe. This happened when she was merely 8 or 9 years old. This painful experience changed her life – and walk forever.

The pain was undoubtedly excruciating for a child that age. What became a more prominent source of danger was the lack of medical care available. Sadly, there was no professional aid for treating Grandmother Betty and her injury in Atlanta during the 1930s.

Thankfully, her own wise Grandmother Rebecca knew a thing or two about removing the poison from the bloodstream. The iron nail infection spread fast in Grandmother Betty's foot, and there wasn't much time to waste.

My Great-great grandmother Rebecca soaked a copper penny in a solution. She then placed it on the bottom of the injured foot, covering it with a piece of salted pork fat. She secured everything in place with a piece of cloth and string and waited for the healing to begin.

To everyone's surprise, the salt and the copper penny drew out the toxins in her blood, taking her out of immediate danger. Several days later, when Grandmother Rebecca removed the pork fat from her foot, it had turned black and blue after absorbing the poisonous toxins from Grandmother Betty's blood.

Without this treatment, Grandmother Betty likely would have died from the poison running through her bloodstream. The old folks at the time highlighted that paralysis would consume her, or she may even develop a disability in a short period of time. Today it is well known that *Tetanus* is an infection caused by a bacterium that often accompanies injuries similar to the one Grandma Betty had.

Every time Grandmother Betty told me this story, she would say, *"That poison would have killed me."* Everyone knew that if her Grandmother Rebecca hadn't known what she knew about the body and healing, we would have lost Grandmother Betty forever.

Although the powerful treatment extracted the poison out of her blood, it did not prevent her from walking with a considerable limp that changed her life forever. Besides the self-consciousness and teasing from the kids, Grandmother Betty had to come to terms with the fact that her life would not be the same.

Due to her changing social life, Grandmother Betty developed a thick skin and a defensive posture to protect herself. Soon, people associated the phrase *"don't play with Betty"* with her. Even though she soon developed a reputation of not being taken lightly, to her mind, the big dream of becoming a singer and dancer was no longer possible.

Regardless of what she went through, she lived her life with humor, style, and grace. She was happy to be alive and always sang and did a little dance for me, which made me so grateful to have her.

Rotten Apples & Witch Hazel

Grandmother Betty used to tell me about a time when my Great-grandmother Lena Mae saved a local girl's eyesight. Although my grandmothers didn't have fancy degrees, no one could compare to what they knew about healing and what I now call *Divine SelfQare*.

It's hard for me to fully recall this story despite listening to it several times when I was younger. I remember how there was a girl in the Atlanta community they grew up in who had almost lost all of her eyesight.

One day my Great-grandmother Lena Mae soaked some rotten apples in witch hazel and let the solution rest for some time. I vaguely recall that there was another ingredient or step in this formula, but sadly, it has been lost forever. However, once the solution was ready, Great-grandmother Lena Mae carefully applied it to the girl's eyes with a cloth. The condition cleared up, and her eyesight was restored successfully.

Spirits of Turpentine

As a child, I remember turpentine or what I now think may have been *"spirits of turpentine"* as a solution for many ailments – most of which my Grandmother Betty directly applied to me.

I particularly remember Grandmother Betty holding a bottle of it whenever I had a stomachache. She would rub some turpentine on my navel and tell me that this would '*kill the worms*' that she believed were causing my stomachache. Another alternative treatment was taking a spoonful of turpentine or likely spirits of turpentine sweetened with a bit of sugar to make the spoonful easier.

Grandmother Betty used turpentine so frequently in our household for treatments that, later, as an adult, I found myself attempting to purchase some too. Astonishingly, I once went to the local Herbal shop asking for a bottle of turpentine because I actually thought that it could be acquired over the counter as medicine.

My dear granddaughters, can you imagine the embarrassment and shock I felt when the shopkeeper enlightened me that turpentine is typically used as paint thinner!

I later read about it in *Medical Apartheid* by Harriet Washington that turpentine was a standard treatment applied to just about every disease, injury, or condition incurred by the enslaved ancestors. To many of our ancestors, this default usage of turpentine was not the most appropriate treatment for every ailment they encountered. They often chose to use herbs and other natural remedies on themselves instead. We will explore this topic more later in this book.

Turpentine was one of the many vestiges of slavery that survived throughout generations of our family. Back then, I wasn't old or aware enough to question the efficacy of turpentine as a treatment, and neither was my father.

In a recent discussion, my father and I discussed how turpentine was a big part of his life growing up with Grandmother Rebecca. To which he said with a chuckle, *"You know Sheila, what doesn't kill you makes you stronger,"* He further added, *"that must have been the case for me because I clearly remember Grandma Rebecca pouring turpentine onto a large spoon with sugar on it and giving it to me to fight off a cold."*

I have also since learned that there is a medical treatment called *"spirits of turpentine."* It is a fluid obtained by the distillation of resin harvested from living trees, mainly pines. Grandmother Betty likely used this form of treatment on me as a child. I am not sure, and neither is my father.

When you read the following story, grandchildren, I want you to know that the women in our family were as courageous as they were insightful about healing. Our ancestors had to deal with so much violence and insecurity that every day felt like a quest for survival. This is a story about how vigilant our mothers and grandmothers had to be to protect themselves and their children when times weren't exactly on their side. As you read further, the lesson I want you to take away is that Divine Health must always be protected at all costs.

Grandmother Rebecca Did Not Play Games

The same night as we compared notes on our individual turpentine adventures, my dad recalled a story of how his Great Grandmother Rebecca lived in brutal poverty when he was young. I was intrigued to learn more about our family's matriarchs, what their life was like, what they did, and how they survived, so I listened intently.

My father didn't say much about Grandmother Rebecca, but the one thing he did tell me is that my Great Great-grandmother Rebecca *did not play any games*. He said that she kept a gun with her when she lived in a multi-unit flat. It was pretty clear that the area she lived in was not safe, which is why she had resorted to keeping a weapon with her that she did not hesitate to use.

As my father narrated this story, I could not help but think how brave she would have been to be able to protect her family and herself in a society so unforgiving. He recollected how, as a child, he woke up frightened to death by the sound of a gunshot one night. As he struggled to focus his vision on the darkroom, he found Grandmother Rebecca sitting up against her chair, with the gun in her hand. He could tell by the smoke releasing from the gun that his grandmother had not hesitated to use it. Someone had tried to break in through a low open window. He could clearly remember the intruder running away screaming, completely regretting entering Great-grandmother Rebecca's house uninvited.

He ended his story by simply uttering the words '*wrong move*', solidifying the fact that his Great Grandmother Rebecca didn't play any games.

Now, my precious daughters and sons, I am about to highlight the most important story that shaped my perspective about the difference between good and evil, the divine and contention. Although I am very inclined to tell you the story, I cannot help but feel how strange it may sound.

Grandmother Betty and the Neighbor

This story is about how a woman poisoned Grandmother Betty out of jealousy when she was just a little girl.

Grandmother Betty once told me that a woman in her neighborhood used a form of spiritual warfare to cause her harm. Back in the day, many referred to this as *putting roots on someone*. As I tell this story, I am aware of how shocking or strange this may feel. Especially to the intelligent and modern society of today, most of you might just dismiss it as a form of superstition or folklore.

However, my beautiful granddaughters and sons, I want you to understand that if you had heard Grandmother Betty retell this story, you would have no doubt about the veracity of the words she spoke. Moreover, how her relentlessness and gift of oral communication made me feel exactly how she felt when she went through such an episode.

When she was young, her mother used to dress her up in pretty dresses and exquisite shoes. Her evenings were taken up by playing with her friends in the neighborhood, and it wasn't uncommon for her to be dressed up to the T.

In hindsight, what her mother did not know was that a woman in her neighborhood, with whose children grandmother Betty used to play, always had a peculiar way of looking at her. While she would play with the children, their mother would eye her in a strange way that a child of that age may not be able to comprehend. Grandmother Betty enjoyed her time with her friends and never paid attention to their mother's behavior; hence, she was never vocal about it either.

One day the woman offered her a cold glass of lemonade. She spoke the words, *"Would you like this glass of cold lemonade?"* to which Grandmother Betty respectfully responded, *"yes, ma'am,"* and gladly took the glass. As any child would do on a summer's day, Grandmother Betty drank it before going off to play with her little friends.

Lo and behold, by the end of the day, she became gravely ill - an illness that would last for weeks. Nobody, not even the doctors, could figure out what was wrong with her. After consulting every possible medical practitioner available to her, Great-grandmother Lena Mae knew she had no other choice than to take her to the local medicine woman. The local medicine woman was a kind and benevolent healer.

The medicine woman, without a doubt, told my Great Grandmother Lena Mae that her daughter had been poisoned. She gave her specific instructions as to what to do in order to reverse the conditions of her illness. With Grandmother Betty's life hanging in the balance, Great-grandmother Lena Mae did exactly what the medicine woman said. You'd be happy to read that her instructions did not only make Grandmother Betty better but, shortly afterward, also helped her discover who put the curse on her to begin with.

Naturally, there was a lot of skepticism surrounding the situation. Great-grandmother Lena Mae did not fully believe that someone could poison such a young child or would she ever recover from her grave illness. However, as time went by, her skepticism began to resolve as, after weeks of deterioration, Grandmother Betty began to heal. The medicine woman knew exactly what was happening and how her patient, Grandmother Betty was recovering. She could predict how her health was going to be in the coming days and how she would recover and begin to get up from her sickbed. Soon, all that she stated happened, and Grandmother Betty resumed her life as a normal child.

With the challenging part over, there was only one issue left to be solved: *Who poisoned her?* As any parent would feel, it was a difficult situation to be in. However, the medicine woman highlighted that the individual responsible for Grandmother Betty's illness would automatically feel compelled to come to their home and check on Grandmother Betty's condition. This would ensure the individual that their poison worked, and Grandmother Betty's death was imminent. But if the individual would discover Grandmother Betty in good health and walking around again, that individual would begin to curse loudly with great profanity and dramatic desperation. The medicine woman prepared my Great-grandmother, Lena Mae, if this situation ever occurred in the future. She said that this particular behavior would indicate the culprit behind the curse or the roots, which meant harm to her family, especially her daughter.

In a short period of time, Grandmother Betty was completely healthy again. She started playing around the house when one day, the same neighbor who poisoned her knocked at the door. By this time, no one ever suspected the mother of the little girls who played with my grandmother of such a deed.

When Great-grandmother Lena Mae opened the door, the woman saw my grandmother in good health, no longer bedridden, and began to curse and yell at my Great-grandmother Lena Mae with the same dramatic desperation the medicine women had predicted. She yelled out horrible profanities in an attempt to spark anger in conflict. But to her surprise, my great-grandmother was already prepared to handle the situation in accordance with the instructions that the medicine woman had provided.

You may be wondering what it was that Great-grandmother Lena Mae did. Let it suffice to say that she utilized divine patience and sacred self-control. It is also safe to say that with the benevolence of the medicine woman and the courage of my Great-grandmother Lena Mae, Grandmother Betty never played with the children of that woman again, nor did she suffer from that illness any longer.

Regardless of how unusual the story might have sounded, this occurrence made me realize one important thing. There is a difference between divinely prepared meals and contentiously prepared meals. The food that you prepare out of love with good intentions brings peace, health, and happiness to those around you. On the other hand, food prepared with bad intentions, jealousy, and underlying hatred always brings negativity and harm. I believe that understanding the difference between the two is so essential that I decided to write about it in my first book called *Divinity Soup: An Ancestor Inspired Recipe Starring Collard Greens* - which hopefully you have read or will read at some point in the future.

I want both of these books to be an inspiration or written guidance for you to be careful about whom you surround yourself with.

As strange as this may sound, you have to keep a check on who is happy for you and who isn't. Grandmother Betty was an innocent child, yet this woman acted out of jealousy. The poison she gave Grandmother Betty could have resulted in her death. Each of you, as my descendants - prayerfully, the future daughters and sons of my own son, should use this book as a guide for life and how to live as naturally and abundantly as possible. I also want you to learn to give with an open heart so that others around you can shine just as brightly as I hope and pray you will.

A Grandbaby's Half Dollar Navel

"Sheila," Grandmother Betty would say, *"have you ever seen people with those navels that protrude?"*

This was a question my grandmother would ask me whenever she wanted to re-tell me the procedure that grandmothers of old used to perform on infants to prevent them from developing navels that extended outward as they grew into adulthood. Recalling the numerous times that Grandmother Betty shared this story with me as a child, I wasn't surprised when she pulled out a shiny new half dollar when I brought baby Zakur to visit with her in her New York City home for the first time.

It was the first night of our stay with his Great-grandmother Betty, and Zakur was still just an infant. In fact, he was probably just a few weeks old. I watched as Grandmother Betty cleaned off the coin with alcohol before using her index finger to gently push Zakur's protruding belly button back inside his stomach. She then covered the opening with a clean, thick piece of medical gauze before placing the coin over it. Using her other hand, she secured the coin in place with medical tape that was durable and safe for the skin.

When she removed the tape a few weeks later on our return visit, his navel was tucked snugly inside, where it remains to this day! This was the strategy that our grandmothers had employed for generations. It was not only meant to be a treatment for what is known as an umbilical hernia in babies after their umbilical cord falls off but to ensure that they had what our grandmothers considered to be attractive navels as adults.

The purpose of retelling the stories that I heard growing up was to give you at least a fraction of the culture and knowledge that surrounded me. Our grandmothers had a strong presence, with their knowledge and strength rising to the top. It is because of their courage and determination coupled with the grace and protection of the Most High that we are where we are and *who* we are today.

I think of the moments where our matriarchs could not or rather did not choose to show weakness, whether it was when they had to hold a gun or heal poisonous blood – they made sure they put in all they had even when the circumstances did not seem to be on their side.

As we reach the end of the stories from the past, I hope that the experiences of our family's matriarchs help to demonstrate that the *Divine SelfQare Strategy* is an essential guide to living, surviving, nurturing, and healing for the future.

Chapter 3

Voice of the Ancestors

Grandchildren, as we continue on our journey to understand *Divine SelfQare*, I am going to discuss in great detail the four elements, **Air, Fire, Earth**, and **Water** or **"A.F.E.W."** Tools. But before I get into the depth of each element, it is crucial for us to gain insights about them from an ancestral perspective.

Just like the stories I've told you about Grandmother Betty and Great Grandmother Lena Mae, there are other matriarchs and patriarchs that may not be directly linked to you by blood, but perhaps by a more special bond – something that ties our entire race together in an everlasting bond.

I cannot emphasize enough how important it is to take into account the voices of the ancestors because they give you an outline of where you come from and the school of thought that they held before you even came into this world. Knowing our roots and stories helps us be who we truly are or become who we are meant to be.

So, now let's discuss the four elements – something that even preceded our beloved ancestors.

The elements have existed on this planet far longer than our ancestors. **Air, Fire, Earth,** and **Water** are four of the primary resources the Most High provided to all our ancestors. With skillful application, the four elements have been a blessing to the ancestors when needed the most. Not only have they proven to be useful for healthy living, but they have also been instrumental in the timeless struggle for freedom.

Ancestral Perspectives on the Four Elements

In this chapter, I will set out to demonstrate how our ancestors not only possessed a specialized form of knowledge about the four elements; but how they even incorporated these elements into their struggle for liberation and health.

Whenever we want to learn about a civilization from the years before us, researchers always take a look at the scriptures, artifacts, or even the drawings on the walls. However, my grandchildren, we are lucky enough to have several inspiring and enlightening texts from our ancestors that help us gain insight into the power that the four elements hold.

> *"It would then reveal to me the knowledge of the elements, the revolution of the planets, the operation of tides, and changes of the seasons."*
> — Nat Turner

It was amazing to realize that our enslaved ancestors not only wielded each element to emancipate themselves from the chains of bondage but also to prevent or cure diseases that otherwise could have killed or made them sick. Through slavery's hardships and the turbulent times of war, our ancestors harnessed the power of the elements to survive. More astonishingly, their literature, speeches, songs, and oral traditions are filled with references to this power. Make no mistake about it; our ancestors were keenly aware that the technologically advanced weaponry of their enemy was what subjugated them. But they also trusted that the Most High did not leave them defenseless in spite of that advanced weaponry. They had **A.F.E.W.** 'tools' of their own:

A: AIR
F: FIRE
E: EARTH
W: WATER

Air, Fire, Earth, and **Water** were found abundantly in nature then and are still available to us now. My beautiful grandchildren, if at any point in the future you should ever find yourselves needing to secure your own health or freedom, I pray you will remember this and actualize the wisdom of your ancestors.

I also hope you feel as liberated and ecstatic right now as I did when I began to decipher the ancestral clues, I'm about to share with you. The statements I have extracted from the speeches, literature, and songs of our esteemed elders will highlight just how significant to us the four elements really are and demonstrate just how integral these powerful guideposts were to our movements.

As I write this book, I feel incredibly privileged to share these Divine Insights with you. My goal in passing down this important legacy of both oral and written tradition is to provide a vehicle for you to inspire future generations to preserve our DNA and perpetuate our sacred heritage.

I will focus primarily on four ancestors, the honorable Frederick Douglas, the honorable Harriet Tubman, the honorable Harriet Jacobs, and the honorable Dr. Martin Luther King Jr. I will also share a few other insights related to some incredible ancestors whose gifts of healing and procuring medicine from herbs during slavery might have been forgotten were it not for the ancestral gift of oral tradition coupled with this book.

This segment will conclude with a quote by the greatest African leader of the 20th century, the honorable Marcus Mosiah

Garvey. In doing so, I will seal this chapter by demonstrating that our ancestors knew exactly what it meant to move through the elements. Let this knowledge from the Most High be a gift that inspires you to think deeply about your culture, environment, and the role you will play in using the elements to keep hope, peace, justice, order, love, health, and freedom alive.

As you continue to read, I want you to reflect on the powerful wisdom conveyed about the elements by our ancestors. Pay close attention to the metaphors they used, as found throughout their speeches, literature, statements, and even in their songs. At times, their words seem like parables carrying hidden meanings - shedding light on a situation or providing answers to questions that could not be safely asked. For to ask, would have been deemed a threat by the existing power structure, and therefore dangerous to the inquirer.

There is also poetry, eloquence, and allegory woven into these parables. Sometimes they are very plain, but the concepts are so out of the normal sphere of everyday experience it may be tempting to dismiss them.

There is always something sacred in the humility of our ancestors. Honor their wisdom and heed their instruction. Many times, when our ancestors spoke of the elements, they did so in ways that were beyond physical – almost *trans-physical*.

Now let's dive into the words of our wise ancestor and patriarch, the honorable Frederick Douglas!

Frederick Douglas Speaks

My sons and daughters, you may not know this, but in 1852, the Ladies Anti-Slavery Society of Rochester, New York, invited the elder Frederick Douglas to give a July 4th speech. The great elder Douglas opted to speak on July 5th instead, and addressing an audience of about 600; he delivered one of his most iconic speeches that would become known by the name, "*What to the Slave is the Fourth of July?*" At one point in the speech, our beloved ancestor proclaimed:

> *"It is not light that we need, but fire;*
> *it is not the gentle shower, but thunder.*
> *We need the storm, the whirlwind,*
> *and the earthquake"*
> *Frederick Douglas*

In this parable, elder Douglas highlights the force required to release his people from the powerful clutches of slavery. These prophetic words eventually manifested in a war so violent that the aftermath was comparable to the devastation left in the wake of a sudden but massive earthquake.

Slavery in the United States was built up like a citadel in ancient times - fortified on all four sides by the walls of economy, legislation, culture, and religion; supported with concrete racism; and sustained by unimaginable violence. Elder Douglas understood what his people were up against. He knew that only something with force equivalent to that of a massive earthquake would be strong enough to topple the foundations that undergirded slavery.

When the elder Douglas spoke this parable, he intended for it to *command* the elements. In doing so, he activated two things simultaneously. He issued a final warning to the United States, and he petitioned the Most High, the owner of heaven and all elements to disrupt the very ground upholding this nation. The civil war broke out about a decade later, and shortly after, the mighty walls that surrounded this proverbial citadel began to crack. The war ensued until, pillar by pillar, slavery finally disintegrated.

The elder Douglas' parable contains all four elements - ***air, fire, earth,*** and ***water***. To understand why one must recognize that the honorable Frederick Douglas himself employed this same wisdom in his own quest for self-emancipation. He himself acquired personal sovereignty by escaping a plantation on foot. Avoiding capture depended on leaving undetected and, at least for some period of time, enduring the raw forces of nature in order to place significant distance and a few obstacles of terrain between him and those who would pursue him.

Luckily, he could secure the help of a confidant, Anna Murray Douglas, who later became his wife, but this type of fortune was unusual. Queen Mother Anna acquired a disguise and secured a boat passage on his behalf, but this kind of escape was not common to most of the enslaved ancestors who dared an escape. As we will hear from other accounts of our ancestors, when sudden opportunities were presented for an escape, they often had to be seized with immediacy. Seldom could they secure equipment, supplies, food, clothing, or shoes. This meant a person could be forced to contend with the brutal forces of nature with bare feet on a long journey north.

Through these types of experiences, our people survived by learning to cloak themselves with nature, to feed themselves from nature, to wield it as a defense against ice-cold temperatures, or to seek shelter in nature's rocky caves during the daylight hours.

The elder Frederick Douglas contended with the four elements during his daring escape. His parable is spoken from experience, not conjecture. He knew and understood that one must take possession of freedom. Therefore, he spoke a parable of warning - like the sound of the thunder alerts the listener of an impending storm.

At one point in the speech, the elder Douglas brings his audience another parable. This time he speaks on the tides of changes that were coming to the nation by focusing them on the ***water*** element. Elder Douglas declared:

> *"Great streams are not easily turned from channels, worn deep in the course of ages. They may sometimes rise in quiet and stately majesty, and inundate the land, refreshing and fertilizing the earth with their mysterious properties. They may also rise in wrath and fury, and bear away, on their angry waves, the accumulated wealth of years of toil and hardship. They, however, gradually flow back to the same old channel, and flow on as serenely as ever. But, while the river may not be turned aside, it may dry up, and leave nothing behind but the withered branch, and the unsightly rock, to howl in the abyss-sweeping wind, the sad tale of departed glory. As with rivers, so with nations."*

To me, the most poignant part of the entire speech was this metaphor: *"As with rivers, so with nations."* This statement foretold the misfortune awaiting a country unable to reconcile with its oppressed masses or predict the level of devastation that was looming on the horizon. The aftermath of the civil war was his astounding proof that just as rivers, nations can dry up and wither too. Here, elder Douglas commanded the destructive or transformative power of water.

This speech makes it incredibly clear that our patriarch, the elder Frederick Douglas, was expressing his will through the four elements. It reveals that harnessing the power of the four elements enabled our ancestors to access their own power. ***Air, Fire, Earth,*** and ***Water*** were more than helpful – they were the tools that gave the weak, overworked, and battered bodies of our people the strength they needed to lift up bare feet and take those initial steps toward freedom.

My sacred grandchildren, do you see? Do you see how the voice of this one ancestor helps us understand the strength and purpose of the four elements? Just like the honorable Frederick Douglas, there are other great voices to be heard!

So, let's continue...

Now, grandchildren, we are going to discuss a parable from an ancestor known for his gift of speech. In beautiful prose, the honorable Dr. Martin Luther King Jr. reveals how the civil rights struggle correlates with the four elements. He even named this powerful force or phenomenon.

Reverend Dr. Martin Luther King Speaks

"Lord, help me to accept my tools.
However, dull they are, help me to accept them."
Reverend Dr. Martin Luther King, Jr.

On the night before his assassination, the honorable Dr. Martin Luther King, Jr. spoke about the experiences of the non-violent movement in Birmingham, Alabama. On this fateful rainy night in Memphis, TN, he described the historic standoff between civil rights protestors and the American government as represented by Bull Connor, referring to it as the *'majestic struggle'* which took place five years prior.

During that era, many African Americans believed that Connor represented the true spirit of the American government. This government empowered him with the unchecked power of a militarized police force that was willing to unleash an army of dogs on non-violent protesters. If this was not enough, Connor was also willing to harm the bodies of the protestors with the destructive power of his fire hoses. Little did he know that those seemingly defenseless protesters had the power of the Most High on their side. They raised their voices in song and, like the winds of a hurricane, drowned out the ferocious barks of the police-trained dogs.

Dr. King's epic speech is one of the first on record to use the four elements as a tool for the expression of the divine passion, war strategy, and self-defense of his people. In one sense, it could be argued that those peaceful protestors were not completely unarmed. Their weapons simply functioned in the realm of the *trans-physical*. As Dr. King articulates so beautifully in the following highlight of what is arguably the most compelling but under-reported aspect of his speech:

> *"Bull Connor next would say turn the fire hose on them. As I said to you the other night, Bull Connor didn't know history...*
>
> *He knew a kind of physics that somehow didn't relate to the trans-physics that we knew about... And that was the fact that there was a certain kind of fire that no water could put out. And we went before the fire hoses.*
>
> *We had known water...*
>
> *If we were Baptist or some other denomination, we had been immersed. If we were Methodist or some other, we had been sprinkled, but we knew water.*
>
> *That couldn't stop us...*
>
> *And we just went on before the dogs, and we would look at them, and we'd go on before the water hoses, and we would look at it, and we just go on singing...*
>
> *Just over my head, I see freedom in the air."*

What makes this statement special and vital towards understanding the concept of this book is how Dr. King refers to the extraordinary ability of African American protestors to turn their experience with the four elements into a tool for self-defense and agitation. Something else to note here is that this speech was orated in front of several sanitation workers during a stormy night. Observing this phenomenon, Dr. King took the presence of the storm and used it to lift the mood by showering inspiration, optimism, and hope onto the fertile minds of his attentive audience.

It is undeniable that Dr. King possessed a gift of oratory. Yet on this particular night, his words demonstrate a deep cosmic understanding of the four elements and the role that they have played for our people in combating both random and strategic acts of brutality and injustice. Dr. King knew just what the elder Douglas understood, and that is the great significance of the four elements in the continuation of our majestic struggle for freedom and health.

Using a metaphoric quality, similar in style, cadence, and power to that of the elder Frederick Douglas, Dr. King introduces us to the concept of *trans-physics* using the elements of **Air, Fire, Earth,** and **Water**. With the precision of a word surgeon, Dr. King proceeds to make the stark contrast between the divine baptismal water that undergirded African American spirituality and the malicious, suffocating water that blasted from Connor's fire hoses.

There is "*a certain kind of fire that no water could put out,*" Dr. King stated, igniting the spirit of divine passion and purpose in the hearts of those listening. This appears to be the same kind of passion that fueled the elder Douglas' intense burning for freedom some 115 years before. Now it was being used to stir up a longing for freedom within the crowd in Memphis, who nodded, clapped, and yelled out words of support in agreement. It should be obvious, but this statement correlates with the *fire* element. This *fire* within the protestors, which no **water** could put out, withstood the bitter-cold blast of rage from Connor's fire hoses. And this same fiery passion enabled the protestors to proceed, braving the bark and the bite of those vicious police dogs.

On the other hand, Dr. King presents us with the **air** element but in a more subtle way. It is given to us through the lyrics of a song. The protestors, seeing dogs, fire hoses, and policemen coming toward them, collectively lifted their faces to the sky, singing in a melodic rhythm, *"...Just over my head, I see freedom in the **air**"* as a source of moral encouragement and strength. Using divine breath, they wielded the **air** from their lungs like a hurricane. This was the force that empowered them to prevail over the fearsome, growling dogs and to persevere through the pain as water blasted onto them from the fire hoses.

When I first heard Dr. King's speech, grandchildren, I found it incredible that I had not given these words much thought before. Now that I am more attuned to the presence of **A.F.E.W.** tools whenever they are presented, I can clearly sense the esoteric way in which Dr. King speaks about the Most High's gift of the four elements. I feel that he and many other protestors consciously tapped into these powerful four elements to rise above that falsehood we misguidedly term, *'white supremacy.'*

In his speech, Dr. King also acknowledged the **earth** element with the metaphor, *'like sardines in a can.'* In this visual kind of way, he illustrates how protestors felt and likely appeared to the onlookers who saw them as they were forced into the back of police vans filled to capacity. Our imaginations were stimulated whenever Dr. King spoke. He so clearly illustrates the correlation between faith, freedom, and the four elements. We can glean from the wisdom Dr. King and the elder Douglas left behind that the elements are powerful tools for us to use at will for freedom. They are also impartial, meaning they do not prefer any one group of people over another. The elements are tools that anyone can tap into and wield for good or evil.

Now beloved grandchildren, can you see how having a firm grasp of Dr. King's *trans-physics* gives an incredible foundation that allows the concepts found in this book to come full circle in a beautiful way?

This knowledge helps us embrace the elements as a tool for liberation against that which ails us. Today, we spend more time-fighting diseases. This fight is vastly different from the political battles fought primarily by our ancestors. Nonetheless, our core message remains the same. We can always rely on nature as a weapon for our self-defense.

For the matriarchs and women of our family who were the true practitioners of Divine Health and matrons of the *Divine SelfQare Strategy*, nature and the elements are the cornerstones upon which our loved ones could always rely. We know this to be a gift to us from the Most High. And so, for us to teach and practice Divine Health and *Divine SelfQare* is like singing an ode to the efforts, struggles, and bravery of the ancestors who fought hard against oppression so that, one day, we could share their wisdom with the generations to come. That's the true power – *Knowledge*.

Knowledge, my daughters, and sons.
Knowledge is Power, hmmm.

Now, haven't you heard this expression before? Well, our ancestors and our matriarchs always stressed the importance of education because it is a person's intelligence that helps them map out their success through life.

Just like worldly knowledge and education, there is another source of wisdom that helps people adapt to, change, or overcome personal obstacles. Many of the oppressed people we will speak of lacked a formal education. They were deprived, overused, and undervalued for the most part of their lives by the tyrants who chose to discriminate against them based on the beauty of their color and nothing else.

But all praises to the Most High! What the ancestors lacked in worldly education, was made up for with the wisdom of *trans-physics,* a spiritual gift that enabled them to wield the power of the natural elements to heal and free themselves whenever necessary or required. Putting *trans-physics* into practice was the extraordinary way of managing the challenges of life using the cards that were dealt to them.

Trans-physics in Practice | Healing Ways and Freedom

Now, grandchildren, you must remember that *ability* is what you are capable of doing. Learning about theories and new ideas may exercise your brain, but truly, it will only really matter when you put your learning into practice.

The kind of *trans-physics* that Dr. King talked about would have no meaning to us today if it weren't for our Queen Mothers Harriet Tubman and Harriet Jacobs, who used their Divine Knowledge to implement healing practices and pave a path to freedom, not just for themselves, but for our race, collectively.

Dr. King introduced the term *trans-physics* to us right before his transition. In doing so, he placed a name on a power we always possessed. Historically, our people exercised power over **A.F.E.W.** tools in pursuit of health, justice, freedom, and goodness. It was used by civil rights protestors to overcome the fire hoses, ferocious dog attacks, and vicious-minded police. This special ability did not originate with protestors from the civil rights era. Many of our self-emancipated ancestors utilized this divine ability to free themselves and others from captivity. No one personifies this fact more than Queen Mother (QM) Harriet Tubman.

Sacred children, listen carefully as we talk about QM Harriet Tubman and how she used *trans-physics* to overcome the hurdles that life threw her way. Immerse yourself in her world and think about what you would have done if you were in her shoes. Draw knowledge from her experience and hold her wisdom in your heart.

Queen Mother Harriet Tubman Speaks

"God's time is near...
he set the North Star in the heavens;
he gave me the strength in my limbs.
He meant I should be free."
- Harriet Tubman

Queen Mother Harriet was known by many titles. To her people, she was a Moses, Deliverer, and Friend. To abolitionist supporters, she was the most efficient conductor of the Underground Railroad. To the US Government, she was a military scout, spy, and cook. To the Union soldiers injured in battle and other sick men, she was a nurse, healer, and medicine provider. To John Brown, the revolutionary, she was 'General' Tubman. But, to her parents, siblings, nephews, and nieces, she was simply a daughter, sister, and aunt. Yet, her enemies called her a fugitive and placed a large bounty on her head. They sought her capture, dead or alive, for doing her Divine Work.

Posthumously, I want to endow her with two more titles. First, I crown her from this day forward, a Master Practitioner of Divine Health. She exemplified the important link between *Divine Health* and the fulfillment of one's Divine Purpose. Second, I recognize QM Harriet's historic and unprecedented mastery of the four elements, and I crown her as the first Queen Mother of *Trans-physics*, for she is a most excellent example of putting *trans-physics* into practice. With her immeasurable contributions to health, freedom, and justice, she showed enslaved people a path to self-emancipation and gave the Union army a strategic advantage over the Confederate military during the civil war.

Although QM Harriet was born into slavery, she was never enslaved in her mind or spirit. The life she lived, though extremely painful, was an extraordinary one filled with humanity, miracles, and unprecedented heroic activity. On the other hand, one could argue that her life was equally filled with trouble, trauma, horrific experiences, and unspeakable suffering. In fact, I would propose that there is a small, misleading dash inscribed on her humble tombstone in upstate New York between the date of her birth and her death. This insulting little dash does little to convey the true magnitude or impact of her life.

The small dash does little justice toward shedding light on her knowledge, skill, and gift for healing and liberating others with the four elements - **Air, Fire, Earth,** and **Water.** The contribution she made in terms of her skills and Divine Knowledge could not be measured in numbers but through the resilience of her race today.

It was her unparalleled knowledge of the four elements and self-discipline, coupled with her faith in the Most High, that allowed her to accomplish what no one else has in all of recorded history. She freed 300 living men, women, and children from the clutches of chattel slavery. For us, daughters of the Most High, there is no debate over the number of people she saved. We are aware, however, that some now propose that we question this number based on the purported limitations of the evidence. In their arrogance, those who do question the number merely insult the integrity of two upright figures in history, namely QM Harriet Tubman and Sarah Bradford. The former is the subject of the book, Harriet Tubman, The Moses of Her People. She is the ancestor who provided the figures, background information, and other historical data. The latter is Sarah Bradford, the author of the book, and QM Harriet's confidant, colleague, and friend. Therefore, the book written by Bradford should be the primary source of all credible knowledge about the life and works of QM Harriet Tubman.

Children, authenticity is everything. If we let our minds become slaves to the media and censorships, we will be practically erasing the contributions that our people made in what was arguably the most difficult time in world history. With the book that I am writing for you today, I am acknowledging and immortalizing the contributions QM Harriet Tubman made through the use of *trans-physics* in freeing herself and people. This zeal, this passion towards our culture, our history, and where we come from is something that I also hope to pass on to you.

The book that I was referring to initially reveals the immeasurable contributions QM Harriet Tubman made to this nation. The depth of her knowledge about the elements and effectiveness of her medical treatments were irrefutable. Her superior survival skills, war tactics, and strategies remain unprecedented. Yet, the world commonly makes the mistake of asserting she received *no* education. As an enslaved person, circumstances and laws made it illegal for her to learn to read, but from our perspective, as traditional healers, and custodians of oral tradition, she was highly educated. Therefore, beautiful daughters, I pray that after reading this book, you will never make this common mistake.

QM Harriet Tubman was arguably one of the highest forms of intelligence during her time, which explains her massive successes serving as a spy, scout, nurse, cook, and 'general' during the civil war. An expert in the field of espionage who often crossed into enemy territory undetected, she came face to face with slave patrols and even the very man who declared himself the owner of her flesh.

On one occasion, she had just purchased food at an open market when she saw him approaching; with cunning skill and quick thinking, she pretended to chase a chicken she intentionally let escape from her grip! This tactic proved to be successful. She remained undetected, safely returning to feed her entourage of the self-emancipated. Her war skills were another constant source of brilliance. She even led three Union gunboats in the famous 1863 Combahee River Raid, freeing 700 enslaved people from a life of bondage on South Carolina plantations.

QM Harriet Tubman's education effectively began when she was afforded the rare opportunity to hone and develop nature skills. As a teen, she was sent to work with her father, Mr. Ben Ross, who made his living as an expert timber inspector. The lumberjack trade required him to spend much of his time in the deep woods, living off the land, navigating through forests, fields, and wading through waterways. He passed his knowledge, skill, and intellectual gifts along to his daughter. Mr. Ross' training proved vital to QM Harriet Tubman, whose career as a conductor on the Underground Railroad was steeped in navigating through thick jungles, rugged terrains, and difficult surroundings.

With her father, she mastered practical uses of things occurring naturally in the material world. QM Harriet Tubman also acquired highly specialized skills like how to interpret the movement of the stars; recognize phases of the moon; predict weather patterns; study the tracks of wildlife, make medicine from plants; extract sap from trees, and identify cherry and dogwood trees in order to use their barks for a wide range of medicinal and other purposes. During this time, she also learned strategies for wilderness survival like foraging for food and recognizing poisonous plants from edible ones. Spirituality and self-discipline were instilled in her by her father as well. He taught her to be an abstemious eater. They fasted religiously together every Friday.

From her mother, QM Harriet Tubman also received a solid education and lessons on how to be resourceful through cooking. Mrs. Ross was the chief cook for the plantation owners and the enslaved. She possessed a vast knowledge of plants, herbs, and natural combinations of these ingredients for food, teas, and healing medicine as well. From her, QM Harriet Tubman developed the skills of identifying, selecting, and preparing edible plants for consumption. She developed mastery in the rich resources of edible plants like sassafras, black cherry, and pawpaw but was keenly aware of the fact that all things green were not safe to eat.

My beloved grandchildren, could it also be possible that QM Harriet Tubman learned from her mother the practice used by so many other enslaved people who dared to self-emancipate, of placing dried Indian Turnip in their shoes or around their feet to throw off the scent of vicious bloodhounds? This was one of the lifesaving strategies that our people used to escape to the North. Since bloodhounds were often used to hunt and recapture anyone who attempted to run away, the pungent smell of this powerful root would help ensure the likelihood of success on their long trek to freedom.

In reality the skills that QM Harriet Tubman developed and honed as a child that transformed her into a skilled practitioner of *trans-physics* were acquired from her parents. These two master teachers, Mr. Ben Ross and Mrs. Rit Ross, both of whom were *trans-physicists*, knew how to safely manipulate the vast natural resources that we today simply refer to as **A.F.E.W.** tools.

As a Daughter of the Most High, QM Harriet Tubman successfully wielded the knowledge she inherited from her parents about the elements to free her people from slavery, ensure the Union Army prevailed, and help heal the sick and dying on the battlefields of the civil war.

> *"She nursed our soldiers in the hospitals, and knew how, when they were dying by numbers of some malignant disease, with cunning skill to extract from roots and herbs, which grew near the source of the disease, the healing draught, which allayed the fever and restored numbers to health."*
> *Sarah Bradford*

An infectious new disease was spreading like a pandemic throughout military campsites during the civil war. QM Harriet Tubman, now serving as a military nurse, combed through infected sections of the camps, tending to dying soldiers, and showing no fear or concern about catching the disease herself. Unlike other doctors in the camp who were at an absolute loss about what to do, she, drawing on previous experience and her encyclopedic knowledge of plants, went to the swamps and emerged with a plan. After acquiring some plants from the swampy region, she began to nurse the men and dress their wounds. Using her special herbal blends, she created teas and poultices that cured the dying men within two weeks of beginning treatment. Once again, QM Harriet Tubman - this time serving as a nurse - prevailed over an obstacle to health or 'swamp disease' using the four elements. Here, she utilized them in the form of plants, heat, steam and tea. Notably, this added another accolade to her growing list of successes.

> *"An invisible pillar of cloud by day and a fire by night."*
> *Sarah Bradford*

Dr. King revealed to us that there was a force operating in nature that enabled our people to counter the racial violence they confronted during the civil rights movement. He called it *trans-physics*. Now grandchildren, do you recall the song the protestors choose to sing at the time of their encounter with Connor and his dogs? The lyrics were:

"Just over my head, I see freedom in the air."

Ironically, this song bears even greater significance to the discussion that follows and is the perfect segue to enlighten us about the Divine Ways the Most High communicated and supported our QM Harriet Tubman throughout her struggle for freedom. On page 17 of the book, Harriet Tubman: *The Moses of Her People,* Bradford wrote:

> *"And so, without money, and without friends, she started on through unknown regions; walking by night, hiding by day, but always conscious of an invisible pillar of cloud by day and of fire by night, under the guidance of which she journeyed or rested."*

Yes, granddaughters and sons, you read that right. Our QM Harriet Tubman, the Moses of her time, was led by what appeared to be an object operating in the skies that communicated intelligently and patiently with her both during the day and at night. She was consciously aware and likely reported to Sarah Bradford that she saw a ***fire*** in the night sky and that it was what provided her direction. She clearly trusted that this ***fire*** was a righteous sign moving in the heavens, and that it was of and from the Most High. She followed it to the destined promised land. She did not omit that the Divine Guidance also provided comfort and direction to her during the daylight hours but this time showing itself as a *cloud* that only she could detect. How do we know this? Because of the word '*invisible*' - meaning only QM Harriet Tubman was supposed to see it. So, is it surprising that few among the intelligentsia have been willing to give full faith and credit to this astounding revelation?

Not to me, sacred children. As a daughter of the Most High, I can relate to having Divine Guidance like this. Many of the experiences I have had over the course of my life, too, defy scientific-based or rational explanation. But, in understanding what Dr. King meant about *trans-physics* being another kind of physics that we knew and drew on from our shared spiritual experiences as a community, this statement is in perfect alignment with our faith and beliefs. The Most High moves oftentimes through signs. What better way for the Most High to guide QM Harriet Tubman, someone already accustomed to reading the stars to navigate through the earth, than by using the very elements she had known and studied her whole life?

Sarah Bradford informed readers of the biography she wrote for QM Harriet Tubman that they might find some of the accounts relayed in the book to be incredulous. She reported that she left out many valuable aspects of QM Harriet Tubman's life simply because she could not find anyone to corroborate them. I think it commendable that she at least included this important piece of the mystery that enveloped our QM's life. It is up to us, the descendants of enslaved people like QM Harriet Tubman, to validate her experiences and affirm her testimony. To say, like Sarah Bradford said, "*I believe you, Queen Mother.*" As I am doing now, and as I pray, you will do once you have the opportunity to read this book and analyze the life story and times of our sacred and most honorable QM, Harriet Tubman.

So now that you've read about her story and contributions, let's examine this statement as Daughters of the Most High with a deeper awareness of the science of *trans-physics*.

First, let's shed light on something important. As Daughters of the Most High, we actively embrace the spiritual principles of fasting, prayer, and self-discipline. We recognize that developing a heightened awareness about naturally occurring events in the environment is a consequence of being in a state of relational intimacy with the Creator. Therefore, we accept at face value, the statement about QM Harriet Tubman being consciously aware of a *fire* in the night sky, and even observing it with her naked eye. Always keep in mind, beloved grandchildren, that our QM Harriet Tubman was a deeply spiritual woman who likely would have heard about and adopted in total faith the scriptural verse in the bible identifying the Most High as 'a consuming *fire*.' We also know this was a real phenomenon to her due to the fact that she either traveled by this force by night or rested securely under its watch by day.

Are you surprised then that the Most High would be with her in the spirit at all times – supplying comfort, support, and companionship during these weary times? Also, note that the Most High did not abandon her during the daylight hours but would manifest spiritually to her in the form of a cloud.

Let's reflect right here for a moment. Can you see it just as clearly as I do? We have once again before us the presence of two important elements: ***air*** and ***fire*** operating in the realm of the *trans-physical*. Therefore, our QM Harriet Tubman was not hallucinating, nor was she disillusioned; but rather, she was both truthfully and transparently sharing her experiences about the elements. The Most High apparently used these elements as a vehicle for communication, to guide, support, and direct a faithful daughter along her very challenging journey.

With these events transpiring in QM Harriet Tubman's life, we might ponder what the source of her power was? On one account, QM Harriet Tubman highlights that she inherited her gift from her father. It has been reported that her father could predict the weather, and he even predicted the Mexican War. QM Harriet Tubman was just as intuitive, knowledgeable, resourceful, and spiritual as her dad. She even had a vision about the end of slavery three years before it actually happened! A testament to this is memorialized in the book that Sarah Bradford penned for her which states:

> *"Three years before, while staying with the Rev. Henry Highland Garnet In New York, a vision came to her on the night of the emancipation of her people. Whether a dream, or one of those glimpses into the future, which sometimes seem to have been granted to her, no one can say, but the effect upon her was very remarkable...The dream or vision filled her whole soul, and physical needs were forgotten."*

Bradford further added:

> *"When, three years later, President Lincoln's proclamation of emancipation was given forth, and there was great jubilee among the friends of the slaves, Harriet was continually asked, 'Why do you not join with the rest in their rejoicing!' 'Oh,' she answered, 'I had my jubilee three years ago. I rejoiced all I could den; I can't rejoice no more.'"*

It was sheer faith in the Most High and confidence in her own ability to utilize and interpret the forces of nature that form the reasons why we can discuss the magnificent accomplishments of QM Harriet Tubman's life today. Just like thousands of ancestors before her, she knew something powerful about *trans-physics* – didn't she? She understood the higher application of nature's elements and used it to assist herself and others who self-emancipated. There were times when nature's presence helped them hide and lay low from those oppressors who sought to recapture them. Even so, QM Harriet Tubman had a wealth of knowledge that enabled her to bring freedom and offer a second chance at life to the people she helped.

My beloved granddaughters and sons, when you read these inspiring events of people who put *trans-physics* into practice, you are becoming aware of who gave birth and meaning to our concept of Divine Health and *Divine SelfQare*. I want you to take a moment and reflect on the sacrifices that our ancestors made for our liberation. We owe our freedom and knowledge to them. Their experiences illustrate how the elements were employed to aid the children of the Most High.

As matriarch of my own family, I hope you, my future grandchildren, develop the courage you will need to become as resilient as QM Harriet Tubman. I truly believe that as a Daughter of the Most High, it is my responsibility to show you ways through which you can help humanity by preaching wellness and becoming divinely led human beings. QM Harriet Tubman's experiences show us how we do not need institutional recognition to be of worth and value to the world.

In the next segment, we will explore the life of a woman who defies easy explanation. A woman whose very determination enabled her to withstand the brutal aspects of raw nature when it stood in between herself and the quest for her freedom.

Queen Mother Harriet Jacobs Speaks

> *"I had never realized what grand things air and sunlight are till I had been deprived of them."*
> *Harriet Jacobs*

Now, pay close attention, grandsons, and daughters, because I want to talk to you about a great icon of history and a constant subject of my studies - QM Harriet Jacobs. Born into slavery in North Carolina, the illustrious QM Harriet Jacobs was just a little under ten years older than QM Harriet Tubman - her namesake. Yet, unlike Tubman, QM Harriet Jacobs actually enjoyed the early part of her childhood - at least up to the age of nine. In fact, when her mother was alive, she had a pleasant childhood. From an enslaved person's perspective, this was not typical.

After the passing of her mother, she lived with 'her mistress,' who taught her how to write, read, and sew. After her mistress' demise, however, she was forced to live under Dr. James Norcom, the father of the young child who now 'owned' her under law. This unfortunate fate proved to be detrimental to both her body and mind.

QM Harriet Jacobs knew the way to freedom was to escape to the free states of the North. By this time, she had two children, who were sent to her grandmother because she was unable to care for them. After planning her escape, several experiences forced her to endure the four elements to survive as she anxiously waited to acquire the help of people who could sketch the path for her freedom.

Sarah Bradford shed light on the experiences that QM Harriet Tubman went through while self-emancipating. Her experiences were different from those of QM Harriet Jacobs'. Yet, we can glean information from both about the challenges enslaved people encountered with the elements on their journey to freedom.

Let's look at a few instances that potentially transpired into examples of *trans-physics* and the higher application of the four elements in a time of need.

> "I suffered much more during the second winter than I did during the first. My limbs were benumbed by inaction, and cold filled them with cramp. I have a very painful sensation of coldness in my head; even my face and tongue stiffened, and I lost the power of speech. ...He returned with herbs, roots,

and ointment. He was especially charged to rub on the ointment by a fire."

In her autobiography, QM Harriet Jacobs wrote about her escape from supposed owners. She describes a series of instances where she had to hide in the bushes, under floorboards, and even on a ship because they were trying to track her down. Through these words, she tells us how she had to contend with the winter to survive. Her freedom came for her at the cost of mental and physical suffering.

You can begin to understand her feelings through the words she uses, such as 'cramp,' 'benumbed,' and 'stiffened.' She lost the ability to move and her power of speech trying to escape. At the same time, we see how a certain individual - her brother - helped her with herbs, roots, and ointments. The use of *fire* in this statement further indicates how the ancestors strategically employed the elements to create harmony where there was imbalance. Here, *fire* was utilized to battle the cold on QM Harriet Jacobs' behalf.

This is especially insightful when referring back to the statement made by the honorable Frederick Douglas, especially when we use it to draw a parallel between collective freedom and personal freedom. The journey for freedom continued for the self-emancipated, even after escaping from the plantation. Keep this in mind when studying our QM Harriet Jacobs' life.

It revealed that even after obtaining freedom and withstanding the perilous nature of the journey; she never fully enjoyed the peace that one expects to accompany the liberated - not when laws and people were put in place to thrust her and anyone vulnerable – whether enslaved or free, back into the clutches of bondage. It was incredible what our enslaved ancestors had to be willing to endure for their freedom. QM Harriet Jacobs endured the following trials for seven years:

> *"I asked myself how many more summers and winters I must be condemned to spend thus. I longed to draw in a plentiful draught of fresh air, to stretch my cramped limbs, to have room to stand erect, to feel the earth under my feet again...."*

When QM Jacobs says 'condemned,' let it indicate for you the great depth of her suffering. She remained steadfast throughout this period of isolation, surviving only on the hopes of a future that didn't require her to serve a life in bondage to anyone. In this process, we witness her transition from a person in total despair desperately longing for a fresh breath of **air** and **earth** beneath her feet to a woman determined to endure all obstacles in order to realize her future filled with hope. This kind of hope expressed by QM Harriet Jacobs can help us cling to the idea that things will get better for those of us who endure through periods of suffering.

The three elements – **air, fire,** and **earth** highlighted in this instance become a form of inspiration because physically, that is what she looks forward to the most. It is almost like she dreams of rejuvenating her body, mind, and soul with fresh **air** and the **earthy** soil so that she can be her own person rather than live oppressed.

> *"In summer, the most terrible thunderstorms were acceptable, for the rain came through the roof, and I rolled up my bed so that it might cool the hot boards under it. Later in the season, storms sometimes wet my clothes through and through, and that was not comfortable when the air grew chilly with oakum."*

This instance is another example of how self-emancipation required our ancestors to contend with the raw force of nature. Here QM Harriet Jacobs highlighted how thunderstorms were acceptable to her because her bed was extremely hot.

The cool rain from the roof cooled the boards under the bed, making her hiding conditions more livable. At the same time, the thunderstorm also wet her clothes and caused her extreme discomfort in the cold.

QM Harriet Jacobs also stated that the rainwater would make things worse as the air grew chilly even with the oakum. Oakum was used as a sealant in ships back in those days to stop air or anything else from entering the cracks. Through this occurrence, she highlighted how the chilly air was able to make her uncomfortable despite the oakum around her.

The next incident from QM Harriet Jacobs' life takes us back to Chapter Two of this book, where we discussed the integral role that our matriarchs played in developing processes to heal and fend off infectious diseases. Much like the narrations about my Grandmother Betty and Great Grandmother Lena Mae, this incident also sheds light on how a 'good grandmother' helped QM Harriet Jacobs get rid of the pain caused by insect bites with herbal teas and cooking medicines.

> *"But for weeks, I was tormented by hundreds of little red insects, fine as a needle's point that pierced through my skin and produced an intolerable burning. The good grandmother gave me herb teas and cooking medicines, and finally, I got rid of them."*

As we walk through different events that transpired throughout history, the role of Divine Health and *Divine SelfQare* via use of the four elements becomes more and more undeniable. Our ancestors knew something about *trans-physics*, something not everyone was aware of, as Dr. Martin Luther King highlighted earlier.

It was this particular knowledge that got them through the hardest phases of life. One cannot imagine the excruciating pain of several insect stings, and had it not been for the healing powers found in nature – there wouldn't have been much to end the suffering. But prior to the insect bites, QM Harriet Jacobs had an even more frightening and painful encounter with nature that could have been deadly for her. In the following account, she explains how a serious injury resulted from her efforts to self-emancipate in the suddenness of night.

> *"Suddenly, a reptile of some kind seized my leg. In my fright, I struck a blow which loosened its hold, but I could not tell whether I had killed it; it was so dark, I could not see what it was; I only knew it was something cold and slimy. The pain I felt soon indicated that the bite was poisonous. I was compelled to leave my place of concealment, and I groped my way back into the house. The pain had become intense, and my friend was startled by my look of anguish. I asked her to prepare a poultice of warm ashes and vinegar, and I applied it to my leg, which was already much swollen. The application gave me some relief, but the swelling did not abate. The dread of being disabled was greater than the physical pain I endured. My friend asked an old woman, who doctored among the slaves, what was good for the bite of a snake or a lizard. She told her to steep a dozen coppers in vinegar, overnight, and apply cankered vinegar to the inflamed part."*

My children, I am incredibly happy to provide you with the knowledge that is supported not only by our modern-day grandmothers but also by the female ancestors dating back to 1813. It makes me proud that the wisdom I am passing down to the generations ahead of me is something that our ancestors have been using long before we even existed.

If you recall, Great Grandmother Lena Mae used copper pennies and salted pork fat as a remedy for a potentially deadly injury my Grandmother received as a child. If you pay close attention, read between the lines, you'll realize how QM Harriet Jacobs' instance of healing is also along the same lines.

In particular, we see how QM Harriet Jacobs was possibly bit by a snake while she was in hiding. Her leg was swollen with reptile's poison coursing through her veins. She asked a friend for a poultice of warm ashes in vinegar to give her some relief.

However, the final treatment was carried out through the advice of a woman who treated the enslaved community with whatever knowledge she had about medicines and treatments. Just like Grandmother Lena Mae, she also suggested soaking copper pennies in vinegar overnight and using the solution to the inflamed wound to draw the poison out.

Yet again, my beloved grandchildren, we can see how most of the women from among our ancestors knew what they had to do in order to survive. It was through their help and determination that many people got a chance to live better lives – free of oppression and free of disease.

The Story Of Sally Brown

As a hopeful grandmother and matriarch to my own family, it makes me proud to tell you stories about resourceful women who also used their *Divine Knowledge and SelfQare Strategy* to better their own lives along with the people around them.

As a mother and hopefully a grandmother to you in the future, I want you to know how lucky you are to be leading the lives you have today. A few centuries back, little girls and boys weren't so fortunate to spend their years in a blissful childhood home. Let me tell you something about a special girl named Sally Brown.

Sally Brown was sold away from her mother at a very young age to be enslaved by new 'owners' on another plantation.

There, she relied on the community of the fellow enslaved people for everything. Being with them taught her ways through which she could manage and alleviate bodily pain.

Sally Brown's story reminds me of my Grandmother, Lena Mae, and how she possessed the knowledge of using copper pennies with other natural elements like food or plants to treat septic wounds. This concoction could treat infections and help alleviate pain from sting bites as well as other injuries. We talked about the same treatment method in Harriet Jacobs' story too!

The existence of the same treatment and healing methods tells us how *Divine SelfQare* has always existed amongst us in one way or another. It is both exciting and beautiful to learn about our ancestors and their ways to heal, treat, and look after one another in a time of crisis. This gift and ability to apply the natural elements to their daily life is what has helped our race survive for so long despite the odds not being in our favor.

Just like the matriarchs of our family have passed down their knowledge to you, the enslaved women became a source of generational knowledge for Sally Brown. Even though she was separated from her mother at a very early age, she was never in the dark about what *Divine SelfQare* actually means. These wise ancestors put *trans-physics* into practice way before us even knowing what it was.

Just like grandmothers, the older enslaved women taught Sally Brown how to use herbs as medicine, something that held more power than a doctor's prescription in their eyes. These women taught her how a tepid bath of leaves did wonders for someone suffering from Dropsy or how using chestnut leaves cured Asthma. Isn't it wonderful to think how our people survived without proper medical care or guidance that the majority of the population is so dependent on today?

I would like to think of myself as a grandmother (whenever that may come true for me) who her grandchildren can approach for wisdom without any hesitation. I truly believe that knowledge is the best gift that you can pass on to children, especially when they have the power to heal and save lives. It was a great source of comfort for me to turn to my grandmother for help, and in some ways, Sally Brown also felt that with the older enslaved women from whom she learned about natural treatments and wellness concoctions.

Using cow manure and mint for tea to treat a certain type of disease, jimsonweed for rheumatism, 'ho 'hound' and sorghum molasses for making candy, Peachtree leaves for upset stomachs, a tepid bath of leaves for dropsy, and for chills - dogwood berries and branch elder twigs, our enslaved ancestors treated their own conditions and fought the disease. But even plantation owners trusted in the root doctors' herbal remedies. The records of many substantial planters confirm how they too took consultation with our ancestors, who were the practicing 'root doctors' of their time.

These healing wisdom traditions of mature enslaved women were nurtured, shared, and transmitted to younger women like Sally Brown. Through this knowledge, Sally had something to develop and nurture of her own. In spite of the unfortunate conditions of being a member of the enslaved class, Sally was the recipient of a treasure. She inherited ancestral knowledge.

My compassionate grandchildren, I want you to imagine how traumatizing it was for Sally to be torn apart from her mother. It is important to look back on our ancestors with empathy and compassion. Yet, this pain and suffering did not inhibit Sally from expressing her love and humanity or seeking purpose in her life. Even through painful circumstances, she embraced every opportunity to learn. Unknowingly, Sally was taught important secrets about Divine Health through *trans-physics*, and daily she developed practical skills for understanding when, where, how, and why to put them into practice.

To fully understand *Divine SelfQare* and the role it plays in Divine Health, you must grasp the concept of the four elements. The elements were often the only tools our ancestors were able to exercise command over to battle the ailments and injuries that constantly inflicted their overworked bodies. ***Air, fire, earth,*** and ***water*** have historically been used by our people to facilitate our freedom and our healing.

The Story of Gus Smith

Now my precious ones, I have another vitally important piece of history to convey about *trans-physics* as revealed through the eyes of a very special ancestor who belonged to that exceptional class of men and women who lived as both enslaved persons and free men. The story of Gus Smith is incredible and relevant. It reveals rarely known, seldom-discussed aspects of our ancient healing traditions. Were it not for this special man, what I am about to share with you would have been lost to history forever. In particular, Gus Smith was the grandson of 'an old-fashioned herb doctor,' a powerful man aptly named Godfry.

Mr. Godfry had the sacred ability to blow out ***fire***, but this was just one among many of the highly specialized skills he possessed. Gus explained that having the ability to blow out ***fire*** meant his Grandfather could completely alleviate the pain associated with burns simply by blowing directly onto the ***fire*** or burned area with the breath of his lungs. Being that he was the only person providing this effective remedy, he was sought after by just about all victims of burns irrespective of race or class who knew of his special talent with ***air*** and ***fire***.

In one instance, Gus recalled when his grandfather treated the child of a man named Charley Stroback whose clothes had caught on fire. The boy had burns all over his body and suffered badly from what was likely to have been second or third-degree burns. No doctors were available who could effectively provide treatment during this unfortunate incident, but his grandfather was summoned for assistance. When he arrived, he blew on the area affected by the fire and in this manner the pain was gone! This skill was handed down from generation to generation to select healers in Gus' family.

It might seem intuitive to you that directing cool air to a burn would bring a victim relief. But this is contrary to fact. Try breathing on your hand right now. Notice the warm air coming out of your mouth? That means the typical person wouldn't be able to provide anyone relief from applying the breath of their lungs to a burn wound. There was something special and unusual about the ability to blow out fire! Gus is describing something *trans-physical* as it relates to the elements of **air**, **fire**, and probably **water**. Whatever it involved should not be dismissed based on what we have learned from our ancestors' wisdom regardless of its probability today.

The wise grandfather knew many herbal remedies that could cure diseases and ailments. He also had very simple ways of diagnosing conditions and diseases. He employed the tools available to him - something common among our ancestors, showing their resourceful ingenuity - to create wellness where there was once sickness and the threat of death and disease. Out of the few herbs that he could still remember, Gus highlighted one called '*white root*.' He mentioned that it was taken out of a bush that grew in the area. The white root was beautiful when it bloomed under the sun but had an awful bitter taste. According to Gus, however, it was known to cure nearly any ailment.

Another illustration of his grandfather, Godfry's resourcefulness, occurred when Gus himself appeared to be succumbing to death due to the deadly typhoid disease coupled with pneumonia. He was so sick; two doctors determined there was nothing more they could do to save him. Unfortunately, at this time, his grandfather was away. But when he got word that his grandson was on his deathbed, he returned, arriving late in the afternoon that day and got to work on his grandson immediately. First, he checked his pulse but could not tell whether Gus was dead or alive from it alone despite still feeling the warmth from his body. So, he asked Gus' grandmother to butter some lightly baked bread and place it butter side down on top of his mouth. The thought was that if the butter melted, he was still living. Gus' grandmother did exactly what his grandfather said, and they all soon realized that he was still alive.

His next step was to whisk a little bit of butter and whiskey together and put a few drops in his mouth every four hours. When Gus gained full consciousness, he remembered waking up to find his grandfather, Mr. Godfry sitting beside him where he remained until Gus could readily identify who he was, then he removed himself fully satisfied that Gus was on the road to recovery.

Other stories of his grandfather's healing folk involved herbal remedies like something he made from an herb called 'remedy weed,' which was a bright green-looking plant that grew around the springs in their area that was used to fend off many kinds of infections or diseases. Similarly, Mr. Godfry employed the use of sarsaparilla root along with cherry bark, pennyroyal, and chamomile root. These, he would gather and then dry out to make tea or a tincture by mixing any of them with whiskey in order to treat a number of conditions his numerous patients presented with.

Sometimes, when a patient suffered from constipation or bowel-related diseases, he reached for laxatives he made from Dogwood buds. Other than this, he had ways to treat sore throats, also known as 'Quincy.' He made onion tea by roasting several onions in ashes, squeezing the fluids from them when done, and having his patients drink this solution as a form of tea.

From these vivid accounts that Gus Smith shared, it should be obvious to you that Mr. Godfry – and ancestors like him - had special ways of working within nature through *trans-physics* and utilizing the four elements. They did so as means of survival, healing, and to secure freedom of the body, mind, and soul from the bondage of slavery, death, sickness and disease.

A Rivalry with Western Medicine

My beloved ones, what I am asking you to do is honor our ancient healing traditions; consider them as viable, research alternative approaches to managing an illness, and create strategies that will enable you to 'own' your Divine Health.

While doing so, I recognize that others may not support your decision; but please do consider this fact. While the doctors alive during the enslavement of our ancestors belittled them for trusting in their own healing traditions and lending more credibility to 'old-fashioned herb doctors' rather than the physicians of slavery's profiteers, they themselves were far from superior in medical training. Most of the so-called physicians in practice during this time only had academic training that consisted of just a few months of medical 'preparation' in a proprietary medical school. So, any suggestion or claims that highlight how these physicians had significantly greater medical training than the practical experiences combined with inherited knowledge of our ancestors are baseless and unfounded.

In fact, many of our ancestor's most effective remedies were often adopted, discussed, published, or even incorporated into mainstream practices or used by the public. Take, for instance, that the South Carolina Gazette published a most effective antidote to snake bites on February 25, 1751. Guess who created it, grandchildren? It was a member of one of our esteemed ancestors who earned his freedom and received an annual pension of one hundred pounds granted to him by the *South Carolina General Assembly* for his tremendous contribution to medicine. His medical wisdom was recognized and undoubtedly saved lives.

I bet you've heard of the Tuskegee experiment that took place between 1932 and 1972. Well, you will be surprised to learn that 200 years prior to this atrocious act against humanity, an enslaved man developed a cure for syphilis! Historically, the records show that an unnamed 'negro man' was paid in manumission with freedom for developing an herbal treatment to cure syphilis. This is documented by a payment made by the Lieutenant governor of Virginia in 1729, who declared that this enslaved man had successfully developed a formula consisting of pharmacologically active roots and bark that proved effective in treating syphilis.

The wonders of our ancestors that relate to healing the body of disease and preventing it from occurring in the first place are seldom known or discussed. Take, for instance, the African origins of the modern vaccine industry. Another one of our great ancestors, whose name was *Onesimus*, is literally the source of one of the most important medical advancements in the so-called 'new world.'

Even so, his face is not painted and framed alongside the celebrated icons who purportedly innovated western medicine as seen on walls of the most prestigious hospitals. Yet, let his name be forever imprinted on the hearts and minds of his own people even though he is not discussed in medical schools or classrooms around the world. But that should not prevent us, as members of his collective ancestry, from calling out his name at every celebration and teaching our children about his significance to health as a pioneer of preventative medicine in the west.

Onesimus should be credited for saving the City of Boston from a potentially deadly epidemic. Here is why. In 1721, Onesimus countered the deadly smallpox disease when he simply proposed a common African treatment to induce lifelong immunity to the disease. This treatment involved an operation that introduced a weakened version of smallpox into the bloodstream or body cavity. Doing so would confer immunity or lifelong protection from the actual disease. What we're explaining here is called inoculation.

He gave this divine wisdom from his people so freely with the hopes of curing the deadly disease and restoring health. This effective procedure brought the death rates down from 14 to 2 percent in a short period. To this point, inoculation had long been the standing preventative treatment for the disease in Africa, but thanks to the work of Onesimus, our African ancestor, it finally became a standard treatment in America and Europe by 1750.

My children, if you find yourself struggling to understand why it is important for you to know, value, and appreciate the power of our ancient healing traditions, trust me when I tell you that these things were oftentimes necessary. To our ancestors, who had no other safe recourse when sick, the sacred power of *trans-physics* as a tool for self-healing was truly seen as a gift to them from the Most High. If you only understood that slavery presented an opportunity for plantation owners to exploit free labor, but it also represents another form of exploitation that is seldom discussed. Medical exploitation is something you need to be aware of, and it is one of the driving forces that compels me to write this book to warn you to take every precaution for your health, whether seeking medical attention for sickness caused by disease or when trying to pursue health proactively through prevention.

During slavery, physicians were just as vested in the system as plantation owners. For them, medicine could not be progressed without experimentation. To conduct experiments that involved high probabilities of death, or which caused excruciating pain, they resorted to using the bodies of our disenfranchised ancestors. For this cause, many of our ancestors purposely withheld information about their ailments or sought opportunities for healing among midwives or herb doctors.

I often ponder over how our ancestors would have survived if they did not have this Divine Knowledge about using nature and all its elements for both their health and liberation. From life and death situations to day-to-day survival, our ancestors, much like the Herb Doctor, survived and helped others around them in situations where most people had given up. If one suffered from chills or related cold or flu symptoms, no problem was without a solution for Gus Smith's grandfather, the ancestor who suggested the use of Butternut Root, also known as a White Walnut, for even the most severe cases.

So, you see, the very lives and well-being of our ancestors necessitated a relationship with the elements that transpired over time into mastery through the healing art and science of *trans-physics*. This took on both practical and spiritual applications for our ancestors, who learned to manipulate the elements through that which occurred naturally in their environment. Whether developing an encyclopedic knowledge of herbs and their many uses or raising their voices in song as they lifted their eyes to the heavens for strength and in search of freedom, the *trans-physical* was born and endured with them through the ages. Now, I am here to make sure that you remember the power and strength of our ancestors. If I have successfully fulfilled my purpose, you will never forget our knowledge, but instead, build on it and cultivate your own.

"I pity the man or woman who has never learned to enjoy nature and to get strength and inspiration out of it."
Booker T. Washington

The Honorable Marcus Garvey Speaks

To sum up this section on the ancestors and their respective insights about the *trans-physical* potential of the elements, I leave you to examine an important statement from the honorable Marcus Mosiah Garvey.

On February 10, 1925, the honorable Marcus Mosiah Garvey wrote the first of several messages to the African Diaspora from the Atlanta Prison after being falsely accused, indicted, and prosecuted for committing mail fraud. Captivating the souls of his people with stirring words and using the same spiritual temerity that the honorable Frederick Douglas employed in his infamous speech just 72 years prior, the honorable Marcus Mosiah Garvey commanded the four elements in the *trans-physical* tradition. Here, however, the honorable Marcus Mosiah Garvey is preparing his people to endure what would prove to be a lifelong mental battle with racism in the form of financial, political, and colonial exploitation. He passionately exclaimed:

> *"If death has power, then count on me in death to be the real Marcus Garvey I would like to be. If I may come in an earthquake, or a cyclone, or plague, or pestilence, or as God would have me, then be assured that I shall never desert you and make your enemies triumph over you....*

...Look for me in the whirlwind or the storm, look for me all around you, for, with God's grace, I shall come and bring with me countless millions of black slaves who have died in America and the West Indies and the millions in Africa to aid you in the fight for Liberty, Freedom and Life."

Chapter 4

Air | Fire | Earth | Water

My children, in the last chapter, we saw the beauty of *trans-physics* in action. Vivid accounts of our ancestors' experiences painted a colorful masterpiece with the ink of oral tradition, public speeches, biographical writings, and poetic songs. Collectively, the words of QM Harriet Tubman, QM Harriet Jacobs, elder Frederick Douglas, Reverend Dr. Martin Luther King Jr, Gus Smith, Sally Brown, and others wove together patterns of health and freedom forming a spiritual fabric that blankets us with protection to this day.

In this chapter, I offer you a brief explanation of the four elements and their relevance in the *Divine SelfQare Strategy*, along with a humble definition of a bold word that sets everything in motion - *trans-physics*.

Trans-physics is the knowledge that always enabled our ancestors to go beyond the obstacles and pain placed before them. By drinking from the fountain of divine strength sourced by the power of the Most High, they emerged from the darkest period in history as *"the world's most enduring and resilient people."*

Consider that on March 7th, 1965, there was an attack on civil rights protesters as they attempted to cross over the Edmund Pettis Bridge into Selma. On that day, an entourage of police officers violently charged toward them with guns, battery sticks, and tear gas.

The brutal encounter was captured in images that circulated the world. The civil rights protestors joined together, collectively uniting based on their inner strength to withstand any outward threats. Were they afraid? I think it is safe to think that some may have been, but they were also fueled by the *trans-physical*, the force Dr. King described as the **"kind of fire no water could put out."** This is where he eloquently references that burning desire that exists within human beings to be free from bondage and many other forms of oppression.

According to Dr. King, having the courage to protest against the forces of racism, brutality, and injustice was not just "*a spiritual experience*," it was "*to be welcomed, even longed for.*"

Now wouldn't you agree that as the children of the Most High, we too should embrace this courageous way of thinking by striving daily to preserve our own health and freedom?

Well, the same burning passion that fortified our ancestors, enabling them to withstand Bull Connor's fire hoses, also enabled them to envision freedom in the **air.** These visions of freedom empowered them as they boldly confronted threats of intimidation, pain, and even death. Towards the end of his speech, Dr. King also reflects on the outcome of the efforts of his people. Through his words, he sheds light on the positive, transformative consequences that result from *trans-physics*, a blessing that proved their collective power.

> "And there was a power there which Bull Connor couldn't adjust to. So, we ended up transforming Bull into a steer, and we won our struggle in Birmingham."

My beautiful grandsons and daughters, Dr. King explained the outcome when he said their **power** was **transforming**. They won that struggle. You must now continue this legacy! In order to do this, you will need to study *trans-physics* and learn to govern yourselves with the *19 principles of Divine Health*. You must exercise regularly, express creativity, uphold morality, and pursue liberty. Now that you have the honor of picking up where the elders, masters, Kings, and Queens of *trans-physics* left off, it is up to you to cultivate your expertise in the art and science of Divine Health through *Divine SelfQare*. You will do this by actively engaging in the daily activities of living, healing, protecting, and liberating yourselves from environmental injustice, medical abuse, and preventable food-related diseases.

Trust me, grandchildren, you should have a solid foundation and knowledge base in order to be a practitioner of Divine Health. In this segment, you will be able to see what it means to be a *trans-physicist*. So, we'll begin by examining the term *'trans-physics'* and defining it in order that you may gain full comprehension of what Dr. King wanted us to know.

Trans-physics Defined

Dr. Martin Luther King Jr., an exceptional speaker of his time, spoke about *trans-physics* with great intention. He combined two important words, **trans** and **physics**, and he did so thoughtfully.

Whenever I want to tell you something, my beloved grandchildren, I give a lot of thought to my words. You know why? Because I understand the power that they hold. What I tell you today does have the power to impact your future, which is why I feel incredibly responsible for the paths you'll choose ahead.

In this manner, when Dr. King prepared his words, I imagine him sitting in front of his desk and thinking to himself about the events he witnessed so many times as he traveled the country organizing marches, boycotts, protests, and sit-ins. He must have thought about the transformative power of **water.** He must have reflected on whether it could be used destructively as when Bull Connor aimed his hoses at the protestors, or constructively, as he himself had done dozens of times by immersing his community in its baptismal waters. He also may have given thought to the *Laws of Physics* and how there was something special about his people that could always enable them to move forward and overcome the most difficult obstacles.

Now, let's break the word down:

The word **trans** is a prefix. It typically means ***across, on the other side,*** or ***beyond***. The word **physics** is a noun. According to the American Heritage College Dictionary, it is defined as:

1. *"The science of matter and energy and interactions between the two, grouped in traditional fields such as acoustics, optics, mechanics, and thermodynamics.*
2. *Physical properties, interactions, processes, or laws.*
3. *The study of the natural or material world and phenomena; natural philosophy."*

When Dr. King created this compound word, it seems likely that he based it on everything we now know about *trans-physics*. The word itself means to go beyond the physical properties or laws of matter, namely, **air**, **fire**, **earth**, and **water**.

Now, my children, doesn't it make sense? When Dr. King noted how Bull Connor *"knew a kind of physics,"* it seems safe to conclude that Dr. King referred to Connor's limited knowledge of matter and how to turn it into a destructive form of energy. Now picture Connor holding a fire hose ready to blast out water. Imagine him as he is honing in on his limited understanding of the science of matter (*water*) and energy (*pressure*). Connor mistakenly thought he could successfully use water destructively to push his will on those seemingly defenseless protestors.

Here, it is very important for you to understand the significance of intent; what you do matters, especially when you do it from the heart. But, if your heart is taken over by impurity, then the choices you make will always cause harm to those around you. The same was the case with Bull Connor. He was a man in the presence of our Creator's *Divine Elements*, he had the power to harness their energy, but he chose to do it negatively. We will talk more about intent and what's in your heart as we move on to the next chapter.

Dr. King also appears to be acknowledging that Bull Connor used his basic understanding of the first rule of physics - but not much more. The first rule of physics provides that *'an object will remain at rest or in a uniform state of motion unless an external force changes that state.'* When Connor directed that water or matter through the fire hoses, he transferred matter into energy. He intended the fire hose blast to be used as an external force against the protesters who collectively formed the civil rights movement. Not only was there an attempt to knock the peaceful protestors off their feet, but to also knock the air out of their lungs.

Fire hoses were never meant to be used on people; rather, they were intended to extinguish a potentially deadly fire. Such waterpower projection could make the person on the receiving end feel as though they were drowning. It also hurt them physically. So how could human beings withstand the ill-used force and survive? This is where Dr. King's explanation comes in:

"a kind of fire no water could put out."

Trans-physics is the force that enabled our people to move beyond the realm of basic physics and prevail spiritually over Connor's mundane use of force. Simply making a distinction between Connors' basic understanding of the laws of physics and our peoples' knowledge of *trans-physics*, Dr. King revealed how the Most High empowered us to move beyond the realm of basic physics and wield its power for the cause. Even today, we can master *trans-physics* and use it for our needs.

My beloved sons and daughters, always remember this essential distinction for as long as you live. It is very important.

Recall that Dr. King made it a point to say that *"Bull Connor didn't know history."* What history do you think Bull Connor was deprived of? I think he was ignorant of the four elements, divine intent, and *trans-physics* as shared through the voices, lives, skills, biographies, narratives, oral histories, speeches, and songs of our ancestors. Could Bull Connor have been ignorant of the historical records left by the honorable Frederick Douglas, QM Harriet Tubman, QM Harriet Jacobs, or the living legacy and wisdom of Dr. King? Yes, clearly this was the case. *Trans-physics* is a part of our history, beloved grandchildren. Own it. Study it. Embrace it.

The significant contributions our ancestors made through *trans-physics* adds a shining star to the endurance of our people. It is due to their historical records that generations were educated beyond school textbooks. Even today, the Divine Knowledge sent down by our resourceful ancestors makes our learning experience outside the traditional classroom wholesome and, more importantly- useful.

We must also honor Dr. King's legacy with renewed energy, strength, and vigor. Hence, nowhere in recent recorded history do we see an esteemed elder drawing a line of distinction in the sand between what we knew and what others knew about the science of matter and how it interconnects. Therefore, Dr. King's name should be spoken with honor, dignity, and admiration. We should express gratitude to Dr. Martin Luther King Jr. for shedding light on the science of *trans-physics*. Without his valuable insight, it is difficult to imagine how we would have been able to add this powerful resource to our *Divine SelfQare Strategy* or use it skillfully for Divine Health.

This ability of our people to survive and thrive collectively is due in part to an extra-physical relationship with the environment as children of the Most High, who relate in very deep and meaningful ways to the characteristics of **Air, Fire, Earth,** and **Water.** If we are to continue to survive as a people living under an asymmetrical power dynamic where technology rules over the masses, then we must equip ourselves with the knowledge of *trans-physics* and use it to defend ourselves mentally, spiritually, and physically. This book and the teachings it contains are like a guide for you to do so, my sacred children. So be vigilant.

We have seen the elements of **air, fire, earth,** and **water** as tools for harm used by those who seek to remain in power through systemic oppression. Consider how these precious resources were turned into instruments of torture and the atrocities committed against our people during legal enslavement. But during this time, we may also bear witness to the exact opposite. Our ancestors strategically employed the four elements to free themselves from bondage and disease with *trans-physics*.

This will only be evident, however, through a deep scrutiny of the stories, songs, and oral traditions of our ancestors. It was these powerful expressions of faith and hope in the Most High, as demonstrated through their life-affirming strategies for healing, survival, and freedom, which explain our reason for being here and as resilient as we are today.

While it may be the case that for some of our people, the science of *trans-physics* was not something engaged in with conscious awareness, it *is* highly evident that *trans-physics* was a clear means of survival for others. We have seen proof of this awareness with QM Harriet Tubman, QM Harriet Jacobs, the honorable Frederick Douglas, and of course, Dr. Martin Luther King Jr. Still, there were others whose knowledge and mastery of the elements, coupled with their faith in the Most High, made them invaluable to our community.

So, my grandchildren, what were the characteristics of the elements, and how did they correlate to Divine Health and equally to our liberation? The key to finding the answer is understanding when to employ each element to achieve the desired goal or a specific result. Whether healing someone of a disease, extracting the essence of a living plant, or securing freedom in the safety of wilderness, knowing when, where, how, and why to employ any one or combination of elements as a tool is our key to success.

Today, if you look around, you will see how the four elements surround your life. It is the *fire* that keeps you warm and kills the bacteria in your food. It's the ***air*** that keeps you cool and protects you from the blazing sun. The ***water*** purifies you and keeps your body running. And lastly, the ***earth*** helps you grow in nourishment with bounty provided by the Most High.

What I am about to share with you will help you gain greater insight into these four elements and how our ancestors collectively understood and employed them for good.

Alright, grandsons and daughters of the Most High, let's begin our examination of **A.F.E.W.** tools.

A.F.E.W. | Qualities & Characteristics

Sons and daughters, our ancestors believed the entire world was made up of the elements, **air, fire, earth,** and **water.** If the ancestors held this belief, wouldn't it make sense that the four elements would also be present in every animal, object, and human? Think about the fact that in the absence of ***air***, human life is measured in minutes. To illustrate the relationship between the ***air*** element and life further, consider that the human body comprises 65% oxygen and 18% carbon in proportion by weight. In reference to the *fire* element, every living being produces heat. The human body even contains a network of nerves near the stomach. Together with the nerve hub, along with myriad arteries and organs, this vast network of nerves reside in a region of the body called the *solar plexus*.

It is called this name because collectively, they look like solar rays. Solar, which translates as the sun, represents the *fire* element.

The *earth* element is seen in the various chemical elements present in the human body. Almost 99% of the human body's mass is made up of six chemical elements: oxygen, carbon, hydrogen, nitrogen, calcium, and phosphorus. Less than 1% account for trace minerals. These elements represent the most basic components or building blocks of all that create the material world or the element of *earth*. As for **water**, it is estimated that 70% of the human body is made up of it, which is a combination of hydrogen and oxygen atoms. Now you see? The ancestors were precise in their assessment.

The ancestors did not only believe that these elements combined with each other to create life in nature and the objects in our environment, but they also realized that when there is balance in the elements combining, only then is there harmony. An observation of the elements revealed to their minds that each one possessed specific qualities. The qualities expressed in simple terms revealed the following:

Air is hot and moist;

Fire is hot and dry;

Earth is cold and dry; and,

Water is cold and moist.

Using this simple but important knowledge as the building blocks of their sound healing practices the ancestors tackled several illnesses. They successfully treated many common ailments and created balance in the body whenever imbalance expressed itself through symptoms of the disease. We saw this with our study of the ancestors who incorporated the elements using the science of *trans-physics* into their sound healing practices.

My beloved grandsons and daughters, do you recall when a snake bit QM Harriet Jacobs during her daring escape? What remedy did the enslaved elder provide for snake bites? It was to soak coppers (pennies) in vinegar and then apply the powdery substance that formed to the wound. This was not hocus pocus magic. The reason is connected to our ancestor's understanding of the temperament of a disease and how to employ the appropriate element in nature in order to bring it back into balance.

See, a snake bite was a lethal injection of poison that caused a great deal of acidity to be formed in QM Harriet Jacobs' blood. Our ancestors would have observed this as an imbalance of the *fire* element. The way to balance acidity is to increase the alkalinity of the blood by applying an alkaline substance (or *earth* element) directly to the wound. Recall that *fire* is hot and dry. They may have reasoned that the remedy most likely to produce the most effect with the least harm would involve an element of *earth*, which we now know is cold and dry. Imagine how our ancestors approached this problem from the logical perspective of a *trans-physicist*. It can be concluded that since the acidity of the snake bite is related more to the production of heat leading to dryness, the *earth* element was the most appropriate element to restore the body to a more balanced, natural alkaline state. Now that makes so much logical sense, doesn't it? Well, let's continue with our study by examining the four elements for their specific characteristics.

Now beloved one, I'm going to talk to you about each of these elements and how they connect to the *Divine SelfQare Strategy* individually and collectively.

Air

When you think about **air**, what comes to your mind? Even though you can't see it, it's always there. Always doing what it's meant to do...Constantly holding you in its embrace as you strive to fulfill your purpose on this planet.

When there is *air*, there is change.

Did you know that it was common for the old folk to say, "*ooohhh child, she changes like the wind*" to describe someone whom they considered to be indecisive or flippy? In *trans-physics*, *air* corresponds with Divine Possibility. The ancestors we have examined looked to the *air* for the source of Knowledge, Instruction, and Guidance about the right way and time to move. We saw this with QM Harriet Tubman, who looked to the night sky for the *fire* element that guided her steps. On the other hand, the day sky gave her the *air* element for instructions of where to sleep while she traveled through scores of densely untamed wilderness situated along with the great distance between the north and the south. We saw it with QM Harriet Jacobs too. She looked to the *air* element to stimulate her lungs and restore her respiratory health after long periods of confinement in the tight space in order to prevail in the psychological warfare she waged against Dr. Norcom, the man who claimed to own her body and soul.

We saw this through the honorable Frederick Douglas, who looked with an unabashed expectation to the *air* for the whirlwind needed to knock out the four pillars that held up slavery in the United States. We saw it with Dr. King through his admission that he and the protestors trans-physically used the *air* in two ways. The first way was when they created a form of directed anti-violence *air* by lifting their voices to sing, "*above my head I see freedom in the air*." And the second way was by actualizing the *air* to exercise Divine Vision, propelling passion beyond one's current limitation. Although we haven't discussed him extensively, we also see it when our ancestor, Nathaniel Turner, a.k.a Nat Turner, the revolutionary who led the August 21st, 1831, insurrection opposing slavery, reportedly stated in an interview with Thomas R. Gray, "*By signs in the heavens it would be known to me when I should commence the great work."*

History records how this ancestor examined the skies in search of signs operating through celestial bodies that would indicate to him the right time to wage war. Lastly, even the ancestor Gus Smith recalls for us the *trans-physical* aspects of the element of **air** by showing us that **air** can be transported from the lungs and transmuted from a state of carbon dioxide into a *trans-physical* element with therapeutic properties. This therapy was used to bring about relief from extreme pain associated with burns and to extinguish ***fires***. Viewing these situational experiences, I think it is safe to conclude that the ancestors interpreted the **air** element as movement, divine inspiration, guidance, and activity.

Fire

Now beloved, visualize yourself sitting outdoors in front of an open ***fire***. Try to hear the crackling sound every time you add a twig to reinvigorate the lighted flames. Imagine the warm glow that emanates to heat your body in the chill of night.

Fire is essential to life, and where there is ***fire***, there is transformation or renewal. **Fire** is typically thought to be a destructive force because devastation and loss can be left in its wake. But beloved, have you ever considered that ***fire*** leads to new beginnings, clearing away the old, and purification? For instance, in the wake of a volcanic eruption, the lava appears as an entirely destructive force that burns away everything in its path. But another way of looking at this fiery essence is through the lens of massive change. Several studies about the geologic effects of lava on the environment reveal astounding information showing how nature and life generally benefit from this process of ***fire*** and renewal. New life is created, the soil becomes rich, the fertile ground enables plants to thrive, and the old dead matter on the ground that operates to suffocate trees and stifle the growth of new plants is removed.

Certain plant species can only regenerate new life in the presence of forest *fires*. For instance, many plants depend on heat or smoke to germinate seeds in the soil or stimulate buds to fruit. Heat-shock can crack open hard shells, liberating seeds or allowing for water to enter. For other plants, research shows a wave of chemicals released by *fire* can pass through the soil, both to fertilize and purge it of toxins. This is the case for some pine and eucalyptus tree species that have evolved into having a *fire*-resistant trunk that can sprout new limbs and regenerate the plant. Most other trees damaged by the devastating impact of forest *fires* actually have to re-sprout from the roots.

To those ancestors who functioned at a *trans-physical* level, *fire* was the chief agent of purification. Not only is it responsible for Divine Activity within humans, but it is also what ignites our sense of Divine Purpose when fueled by our faith in the Most High. You may not have paid attention to this before, but phonetically, the word '*Fire*' can be heard whenever someone utters the word '*Purifier*.' We enunciate it as '**Pure-e-Fire**.' Can you hear it? Perhaps to some people, this is just coincidental, but for us, it is more of a spiritual clue to pay attention to the cleansing properties of *fire* and the conditions that create it. Whatever the case may be, my divine grandsons and daughters, it is on point and par with our concept of *trans-physics*.

Fire as an element equipped our ancestors with power and opportunities to transcend the realm of stagnation, oppression, death, slavery, and disease. Dr. King brought awareness to this concept when he stated, "*there is a kind of fire that no **water** could put out*." This type of *fire*, the one Dr. King refers to, does not damage those who behold it or harm those who find themselves in its presence. It is not seen with the naked eye. It only exists spiritually. Yet, it is felt within every human being and is a driving force that constantly or periodically motivates us to do something, such as taking calculated risks or bringing something from the unseen realm of ideas into Divine Reality. I have heard Dr. Myles Munroe, the profound teacher of *Kingdom principles*, refer to what I am speaking about with a scripture from the bible that provides:

> *"And I will give unto thee the keys of the kingdom of heaven: and whatsoever thou shalt bind on earth shall be bound in heaven: and whatsoever thou shalt loose on earth shall be loosed in heaven."*
> Mathew 16:19

Thus, we can relate this to QM Harriet Tubman, who, in her quest to *"loose"* herself and her people from bondage on **earth**, is likely to have *"loosed"* something of equal magnitude in heaven. For the faithful, it was clearly the much-needed help of the Most High. To her sons and daughters in the spirit, it is plain to see that the Divine One moved with her as that *"invisible **fire** by night."* It was the Most High who provided this invisible **fire** and guided her through unknown territories. Our ancestors experienced this type of **fire** whenever it was time to heal, inspire, and summon the courage required to escape bondage. My beautiful granddaughters and sons, you too have the power to transform reality. Begin to purify your own thoughts and acquire knowledge, wisdom, resources, and power.

Earth

Now my children, where there is **earth**, there is an abundance of life. Everything from the blooming flowers and evergreen trees we see, to the wild cherries and fresh produce I hope to cook for you one day is a work of art. The Most High is the master artist, and all life on **earth** is an expression of Divine Beauty and creation. The **earth** is blessed. And like a blank canvas, the ***earth*** is filled with the beautiful hues we call life by the Most High.

There is evidence of this fact in the plants, animals, microorganisms, sea creatures, and human beings who reside and rely on the ***earth*** in the fullness of its abundance. Our ancestors typically equated the ***earth*** element with the feminine qualities of creativeness, gradual change, motherhood, fertility, nurturing, caring, and giving. ***Earth*** is grounding and provides a stable foundation upon which all human ingenuity and efforts can be laid. The cradle of civilization is a euphemism that leads to the idea of the ***earth*** being associated with pregnancy, birth, and motherhood. Naturally, all origins date back to our ancestors who first occupied the ***earth*** on the most abundant continent today and then - Africa. ***Earth*** is connected to the infinite as a divine part of creation. It is one of the few planets in our known galaxy that houses all the elements essential for human, animal, and plant life. It is an atmosphere that creates a form of biodiversity and evolves to accommodate internally and externally induced factors that lead to change.

To our ancestors, who mastered the art and science of *trans-physics*, the ***earth*** element was a tool for creating the conditions to build, sustain, and improve life. QM Harriet Tubman illustrates this best with her use of plants to secure medicine to treat deadly swamp diseases. Swamp disease was a consequence of being out of harmony with the ***earth***. It created sores and rashes and exposed the skin to deadly infections, along with high levels of heat in the body that we refer to today as a fever or temperature. The remedy was near the source of the disease. As a *trans-physicist* with access to Divine Knowledge, QM Harriet Tubman knew how to address this expression of illness.

The honorable Frederick Douglas knew what the honorable Marcus Mosiah Garvey knew, and what so many others knew, that the ***earth*** element is aligned with the courses of freedom and justice. They understood that in the presence of the most extreme forms of human exploitation, the power potential within the **earth** might be your best tactical defense or offensive ally. Elder Douglas reminds us that the **earth** has a quake potential that can generate a weapon, and together, working in coordination with the other forces of nature, circumstances can help subdue the enemy. Ironically, both these ancestors saw the **earth** and other elements as tools for destroying oppression and petitioned the Most High, as the Creator, the Protector, and the Ultimate War Strategist, to employ them for that purpose.

Water

Think about **water** trickling down your skin. This sensation should crystallize for you that whenever *water* is present, there is movement.

This is because *water*, among its many functions, serves as a vast transportation system. In humans, *water* carries vital nutrients throughout the cells. In the *earth*, *water* moves above, through, and beneath the ground to create and sustain life. *Water* is known as the universal solvent. It can dissolve practically any substance over time. Without *water*, neither our bodies nor the *earth* could regulate temperature efficiently. In fact, our kidneys and all other organs require *water* to work. *Water* is key to healthy skin, cleansing and removing toxins from the body through sweat, urination, and even mucous.

When QM Harriet Tubman needed a safe passage through the wilderness to freedom on many occasions, she and her company waded through the *water*. When the honorable Frederick Douglas commanded the elements to overpower slavery, he demanded that thunder and lightning replace the gentle *shower*. When Dr. King and his group of peaceful civil rights protesters confronted the violent use of **water** projected through **fire** hoses, they were keenly aware that it was meant to move them out of their position and knock them off their stance of moral supremacy. Yet, they drew on their collective experiences with *water* as a gentle force that moves the spirit into the realm of possibility with the Most High and Dr. King stated:

> "We had known water. If we were Baptist or some other denomination, we had been <u>immersed</u>. If we were Methodist or some other, we had been sprinkled, but we knew water. That couldn't stop us...."

I hope I have opened your mind to the idea that the ancestors had a deep relationship with the elements. This relationship extended beyond the *Laws of Physics* into the higher ways of thinking and knowing about the world and a vast array of resources through their knowledge of *trans-physics*. To this extent, our ancestors formed healing traditions on the four fundamental characteristics of the elements.

As I highlighted to you previously, my sacred grandchildren, these traditions were based on the simple building blocks of wisdom demonstrating that **air** is hot and moist, ***fire*** is hot and dry, the *earth* is cold and dry, and *water* is cold and moist. Using this observation, they were able to address many aspects of life, including the foundation for developing and administering herbs and roots as medicine, as well as, securing their freedom.

This chapter was meant to shed deeper knowledge and awareness of **A.F.E.W.** tools, a term I coined while defining the art and science of *Divine SelfQare*. It should express to you how our ancestors employed the elements in a conscious manner to articulate effective healing strategies.

Experts state that when a person is demoralized, they often lose their ability to assess true information. As a result, such a person may refuse to believe the truth of his own power and greatness. During the last 400 years, the ancestors and their descendants experienced an entire system of demoralization, *a type of psychological warfare* in an effort to change their perception of reality. That is why I am compelled by the divine force that defines my relationship with the Most High to write this book.

These are the metaphorical keys to Divine Health. Today, I give them back to you. We always had them, but through the turbulence of the times, we nearly lost them again. The four elements help us in a myriad of ways to overcome the obstacles we face. Not only are they available for you to use freely, but they are also vital to our work as practitioners of Divine Health. Use them for higher applications such as the facilitation of *Divine SelfQare*, and when necessary to survive life's many challenging circumstances. More than several of our ancestors have *awed* mankind with the most basic application of these elements at different points in time. I pray that you will do many great things with them too.

As you continue reading along, there will be a point in this book when I teach you how to utilize these elements personally for your *Divine SelfQare* and Divine Health Journey. But for now, the next task is to grasp the one thing that binds all our work as Divine Children of the Most High. That is, you must now understand what it means to have and master the fifth element, which is Divine Intention.

Chapter 5

Fifth Element | Divine Intention

My beloved granddaughters and sons, I have come to a point in this book that deals with a matter of great consequence - a matter that concerns all human interactions and governs all human behavior. It addresses the unspoken concerns of human nature as often it is concealed within the heart or chest of every human being. Whether innocent or wicked, what I am speaking about is *intention*. Whether good or bad, indifferent or altruistic, a person's intentions will dictate their actions and eventually reveal the truth through its consequences.

But, as I write this section of the book, grandchildren, I cannot help but ponder on all the beautiful lessons I've learned from studying our direct and collective ancestors. I also reflect on my meditations and insights from the ultimate teacher, the owner of consciousness - the Most High, as well. The beauty of this chapter of our journey together through time is that I get an opportunity to share wisdom with you about the importance of the fifth element, *Divine Intention*.

I have previously discussed the phenomenon used by our ancestors to provide the best and most appropriate intervention for each challenge they faced in an effort to overcome sickness, injury, slavery, and other personal and collective obstacles to life. It was through the science of *trans-physics*.

As a mother and, more importantly, as a daughter of the Most High, I express my love in many ways. One way is by helping each of you identify with and find dignity, power, and hope in the heroic, brilliant efforts of our resilient ancestors, whom we've discussed so far—those who wielded the elements for health and freedom.

The literary works of our ancestors, when read collectively as inter-texts, reveal a complex understanding of both physics and *trans-physics*. This knowledge and its application enabled them to engage the four elements as potent tools for liberation, health, and disease prevention. However, the truth of the matter is that nothing happened *trans-physically* without the Fifth Element.

To answer your question about why intention matters, my precious children, Divine Intention is what marries the science of *trans-physics* to the art of healing and liberation using the four elements. What makes intention so important is that it is difficult to detect in the cunning and ruthless. The very nature of *intention* is deeply connected to four novel concepts, which I will highlight ahead.

You might be curious as to why this lesson is of such massive importance to your grandmother. I wish for you to know this as well. If I had access to the important information that I am about to share with you when I was young like you are now, it would have spared my body, mind, and spirit many hardships. Some of these hardships I speak of were things I endured as a consequence of naiveté. See, there was a time when I believed that people always meant what they *said* and behaved in ways consistent with their *beliefs*. But that was not true. Trust me, children, your wise grandmother is about to teach you about things that can save your life if understood fully. So, take heed now to the lessons that follow.

My sacred granddaughters and sons, I hope this powerful wisdom will help you see that *Divine Intention* is the force that generates the power behind the science of *trans-physics*. It does so by bridging the gap between human conduct or (seen) behavior and the *(unseen)* spiritual nature of intention. Now, I want to take a moment to provide insight about *Divine Intention* specifically and reveal other forms of intention as well.

As you read the following four stories, think about the ways in which people in the story interact; how they *initially* present themselves; and, whether their behavior is *consistent* throughout. Observe whether the perception you have of these people at the beginning of the story contrasts with how you think about them at the end. The questions that should rise are: *what was their true intention,* and *was the intent they expressed toward the end of the story in alignment with their behavior at the beginning of the story?*

Note what behaviors they employ as they set out to achieve their end goals. You may recognize some qualities and characteristics in yourself or others that you know - traits that disturb, resonate with, or inspire you based on your own experiences with life. Embrace and, if necessary, document those feelings so that later you can reflect on why.

Before we begin, I want you to know that these stories are close to my heart and that sharing them with you makes me truly value my role as a bestower of Divine Knowledge as I inherited from the generations before me.

My goal in writing this is to instruct you about the nature of people in the world so that you will be equipped in all ways to manage them. With the purity in your hearts and the sound wisdom of your minds, you will shine like a beacon of light in the world and help to guide others. Let's begin...

Clean Face | Pure Heart

When I was a little girl, I remember one rare occasion when I accompanied Grandmother Betty on the subway to Times Square to meet her friend, Mr. Cecil. Believe it or not, Mr. Cecil was a professional panhandler, meaning he made his living simply by requesting money from the people who passed him by on their way to work, shopping, or even from tourists. Mr. Cecil was never viewed negatively for his work. There was real dignity in Mr. Cecil. He had not been in this position his whole life. Before an unfortunate series of events caused him to go blind and suffer from paralysis from the waist down, Mr. Cecil enjoyed a bustling life of independence and full mobility.

In fact, he knew my grandmother from her youth. He dated her for many years. They remained friends even after the courtship. So, Mr. Cecil knew if he could trust anyone with life, it was his old confidant and friend, my grandmother, Betty. When we arrived, I saw the man I had heard about my whole life. There he was, cup in hand, warmly dressed and looking a little bit unkempt - as you might expect of a man stricken with his condition to appear. But what I noticed is that he spoke to the people who stopped with a great deal of interest and familiarity. *"How's it going today, Cecil?"* One man would ask him while folding a bill of money and placing it into the cup. Then someone else zipped by, quickly tossing a coin or two into the cup, yelling, *"Hey Cecil, see you tomorrow! Gotta run, I'm late for my appointment,"* his voice fading as they moved further and further away. Using his raspy voice, Mr. Cecil would respond to both by their first names. He recognized all his friends' voices.

This kind of concerned exchange went on for almost an hour as my Grandmother, and I stood by him watching. At one point, Mr. Cecil finally addressed me, even introducing me to one of his other close companions. He said, *"Glad to finally see you, Sheila,"* with a hearty chuckle and then reminded me that we weren't strangers since we had spoken over the phone many times. Even to me, it didn't seem like our first time meeting up. He shared how he'd kept up with my grades and school performance through my grandmother over the years. There was no doubt in the fact that Mr. Cecil was a kind soul.

After a while, we headed back to his apartment. He lived in a small flat in Manhattan that had a little bit of furnishing, a twin bed, and television that he listened to for the news and entertainment, along with a few dishes and eating utensils that were in the sink needing to be washed. My grandmother's job was to count all the money, tell him how much he earned, and place it inside his special envelope. She would also help him make payments to his utilities and obtain some groceries for a few days after tidying up the place a little. For this work, he would give her a reasonable portion of his earnings.

The two had this mutual trust and confidence in each other developed over decades. My grandmother unfolded each bill, spreading them over the table as she counted each one aloud for him to clearly hear her as she carefully placed each bill onto the palm of his outstretched hand, stacking the bills from smallest to biggest. Then she counted the coins. This ritual they shared with each other over many decades until the day Mr. Cecil died; always without incident or distrust.

Some income days were better than others, but Mr. Cecil made his way in the world, supplementing what little governmental benefits he received from panhandling. Mr. Cecil made me realize that panhandling is not begging under the circumstances like his. It was a form of income earned through speaking to people developing a relationship of genuine, mutual concern with folks on a daily basis. These folks were genuinely interested in him as well. They admired him for having the courage and will to get up and try day after day.

Grandmother Betty and Mr. Cecil's relationship demonstrates that aspect of **Divine Intent** whose attributes will be known to you from this day forward as *clean face | pure heart*. They trusted one another and honored their friendship. Together they worked to ensure that one another's basic needs could be met honestly. The people of Times Square trusted and cared for Mr. Cecil too. Seldom did anyone who knew him ever attempt to harm, cheat, or rob him of his earnings each day even though he may have received a large sum of cash. His community protected him. There was respect for the humanity of individuals back then, and it didn't matter what the person's circumstances were.

My precious grandchildren, you must ponder on the actions of our Queen-Mother and matriarch, Grandma Betty. It is important to understand that her conduct being a woman of upright character expressed as **Divine Intent** is part of the attribution that I want you to think of from here on as *clean face | pure heart*. For now, suffice with what I have shared and read on.

The next story is equally important for reasons I believe will become apparent to you. It is a story meant to illustrate wicked intent, which is the opposite of **Divine Intent**. So read along now, my love.

Clean Face | Impure Heart

Julissa met Michael at a local networking event for aspiring entrepreneurs. They realized after a brief discussion that they had so much in common, but best of all, they both had skills, resources, and ambitions that complemented one another. As they continued their discussion over the course of a few weeks, they recognized that going into a formal partnership could help boost themselves as tech executives by filling in each other's gaps. Julissa had a real estate property that wasn't being used and costing her because, after the three-month pandemic, she couldn't afford the repairs. Michael had a list of contractors who would gladly barter their services in exchange for some office rental space. It was a match made in heaven.

Julissa was so confident in Michael that she disclosed some matters about her personal life to him. In particular, she revealed that she was having trouble with her son, Drew. She confided a great deal related to the problems she was having with Drew. Divulging how he had gotten involved with some kids who were engaging in risky behaviors. Just discussing her life with Michael was one thing that bought her a sense of peace because she was worried that Drew wasn't just a recreational user anymore. She thought that he was beginning to sell marijuana.

The recreational use of marijuana was illegal in the state of Maryland. When Julissa shared this information with Michael, he assured her that everything would be okay. She just felt safe when talking with him about her life. She felt that she could always trust him, and he generously encouraged her to keep him abreast of anything going on in her life, whether by text or phone; he was always there. Julissa felt comforted by this kind gesture.

After a while, the partnership blossomed. The tech incubator was attracting new innovators and making money from both rental income and helping to patent and trademark great concepts from start to finish. After one year of success, Michael and Julissa decided to change their partnership terms to anticipate more growth. But, Michael presented Julissa with a one-sided contract. Under the new agreement, he would take majority ownership of both sides of the company, leaving Julissa with only a 30 percent interest in just the rental income! She would hold no ownership interest in the venture capital side of the company!

Julissa was appalled and insulted, but before she could curl her lips to give him a piece of her mind or inform him that she would be calling a lawyer, Michael quickly reminded Julissa to consider all that he knew about her son's *recreational* habits. Hence, his offer was more than generous.

Michael spoke to her with an antagonizing tone that Julissa had never heard. He went on to speak about Drew as being a criminal, about how even recreational marijuana usage was illegal in Maryland and remarked to her that Drew was now clearly addicted to the marijuana that he *sold*. He spoke in a very wisenheimer way about how unfortunate things could turn out for her and Drew if he were convicted of marijuana possession and, worse - its distribution.

With shaky hands, swollen eyes, and tears rolling down her face, Julissa signed the ruthless, unfair contract, reluctantly giving up her fifty percent interest in the two lines of business. She felt she had no choice but to accept a mere thirty percent interest in the rental income alone. She did so after a quick but careful analysis of the misfortunes that would befall her and her only son if he were to be labeled a 'drug dealer' or criminal. Plus, she knew that any harm to her reputation would severely diminish future business opportunities with prospective clients - she simply could not afford the scandal at this time. So she signed part of her life away.

You see, children, Julissa experienced what shall be known to you as *clean face | impure heart*. Trust me, my grandchildren, I will explain later. But for now, as you ponder the events that transpired in this story, I want you to reflect on Michael's behavior throughout the story.

Would you agree with me that Julissa grossly misunderstood Michael's ambitions, character, and intentions? I mean, isn't it clear to you now that although Michael seemed like a friend with his big, toothy smile, calming voice, charm, and gentle disposition, this *face* that he put on led Julissa to underestimate him? Julissa's mistake was understandable; he always presented himself to the community as someone who could be trusted. She thought of him as someone who cared about her and who had her best interest. Julissa learned the hard truth about a phenomenon known as a *clean face | impure heart*.

Now, let's move on to the next topic, *unclean face | pure heart*.

Unclean Face | Pure Heart

One day, a beautiful summer day, a young lady began her daily walk down the street to retrieve some lunch from her favorite food spot when she spotted a homeless man. Feeling generous, she stopped in front of him as he sat on the concrete sidewalk in front of her office building. Pulling out a dollar and a few coins, she cheerfully dropped them into the cup that he held up towards the money in her hand. With a deep sense of gratitude and a smile, the man thanked her in his big voice.

She smiled at him and kindly whispered sweetly, *"you're welcome."* When she got home and started to unwind later on that evening, she decided to wind down with a warm bath. As she went to remove the engagement ring from her hand in order to secure it safely on the counter so she could bathe, much to her trepidation, the ring was not there! It was not nestled snugly on the fourth finger of her left hand where it was this morning when she went to work!

Her long-standing boyfriend, Ron, had just surprised her a few weeks ago at an engagement party with the ring as she stood there speechless, crying tears of joy while completely surrounded by family and close friends. As memories of that special day filled her mind, she began to feel overcome with grief and began to cry. The loss of this precious gift was a lot to bear. How could she tell her fiancé? Just as she pondered the thought, her best friend, Kim, happened to call. Together on the phone, they tried to retrace her activities for the day. Instantly they came to the same conclusion! The ring had to be in possession of the homeless man - the one she helped earlier that day.

They decided it was too dangerous to go looking for the homeless man after dark, but first thing in the morning, they both would check to see if he showed up at the same spot. When the two women approached the location, they were shocked to find that he was still there. As they approached him, the homeless man put a big smile on his face. He knew exactly why the woman had returned. Before she could open her mouth, the man lifted his eyes and extended his hand toward the woman. Between his index finger and thumb was the beautiful diamond ring still glistening. The woman once again began to cry as she thanked him repeatedly.

All the commotion attracted the interest of the people passing by, and eventually, a small crowd formed around the three of them. People applauded and shed tears of their own as they began to hear about the astonishing story of how a homeless man blessed a woman who thought she was blessing him. The local news got wind of the story and interviewed them both the next day. When the reporter asked him why he returned the ring, the homeless man said that he knew how important the ring must have been to the woman and remained in the spot the whole night, hoping that she would come back. The homeless man illustrates the third attribution or way of exposing one's true intent known as *unclean face | pure heart*.

Lastly, let me shed some light on *unclean faces and impure hearts*.

Unclean Face | Impure Heart

On October 12, 1492, the lives of King Guacanagari, his chiefs, principal men, and people changed forever. The graphic accounts of what happened to the Taino people after meeting the Spanish explorer, Christopher Columbus, can be found in a book published by Bartolom de Las Casas in 1542 titled, *"A Short Account of the Destruction of the Indies."* But what might King Guacanagari say about the events leading up to the ultimate ruin of his people if he could speak directly to us today? What would he want us to know about the many atrocities suffered by the Taino under the eye of Columbus?

We may never know for sure, but the following story is meant to portray a lesson to you about *unclean face | impure heart*, the fourth and final attribution of intent. As a reader, you will find yourself in the shoes of King Guacanagari - to give you a better understanding of how he may have felt during his encounter with Columbus, whose agenda and crew, both, unfolded before his eyes.

As you read the following narrative, imagine it as historical fiction and use your Divine Imagination to visualize what it must have been like for the Taino people to experience the brutal exploits they suffered at the hands of Spain's colonizers. This kind of brutality would become the hallmark of their Queen's colonial power over indigenous people around the world.

Continue reading, beloved, because even today, the world is full of Columbuses, and therefore, this is an important concept for you to grasp. This means there is a high likelihood that at some point in your life people will show up with cruel intentions. These people will desire to exact suffering from you or bring strife into your life. People *will* come with *unclean faces | impure hearts*. Most will be expecting you to be ill-prepared.

Hopefully, after reading this book and arming yourself with its wisdom, you will be ready to face them in all the ways they like to present themselves. That is, if I have accomplished my goal as a grandmother, great-grandmother, and thoughtful matriarch. Time is of the essence beloved; continue reading because the story begins now...

> *As difficult as it is to imagine now, more than 600 years ago, this land was populated with hundreds of thousands of people. People who belonged to many nations that were indigenous to this great land. Among them were my people, the nation of*

the Taino, and I, King Guacanagari, ruled them justly.

Together we enjoyed the bounty of nature, lived off the great abundance of the earth, feasted from the vast provisions of the land, and coexisted in peace and harmony with nature as we had done seamlessly for countless generations. But, when I reflect on the period of my reign as King of the Taino people and the events that ultimately led to our destruction, I am overcome by great sorrow.

In many ways, I failed my nation. I ignored the signs and prophecies that warned me of the great and terrible times when terror and tribulation would befall my people. I was disarmed by my own curiosity and desire to be recognized by foreign rulers. I did not heed the advice given to me by those great sages of my nation who offered guidance about Columbus and his far away Queen. I even dismissed the council of twelve elders. These wise women cautioned me not to be careless about my interactions with the foreign explorers. They told me about what terrible things they saw in the restless eyes of these men.

They saw betrayal.

They warned me that when Columbus spoke, he did so in the manner of the rattlesnake, with a forked tongue. Yet, in spite of all their spiritual guidance and wisdom, I had more confidence in my own beliefs about the men who arrived at our shores in those large water vessels.

I confided in and trusted Columbus. Unlike the elders, I did not find cause to think of him as suspicious. He seemed to pose no threat at the start. The strange ways in which he and his comrades spoke, dressed, and behaved with each other, induced me to let my guard down. I thought very fondly of them at first. But this, too, would prove to be one of numerous mistakes I made.

Lending my trust to these foreign men proved to be my greatest mistake. Therefore, it is with deep shame and even deeper regret that I convey these harrowing accounts to you. Trust me; I am filled with pain as I relive the events that destroyed my people. Yet, I endure the pain anyway, so others may learn from my life's lesson. This is something you need to know...

*This tragic saga began on what seemed would be any other ordinary day in our lives. As Taino, we organized our life work according to the seasons, and this was the season of momentous change. A time when the forests would change from vibrant evergreens to an array of red, orange, and brown leaves. I never thought that this sign would be the first indication of my failure, a spark that would ignite the **fire** of destruction like a reign of terror - one that would eventually set the entire world ablaze and cause massive change. The cost would be the loss of millions of lives to extinguish the light of eternal happiness for millions more here on these shores and around the world.*

A few hunters returned to the village earlier than usual, but instead of buffalo, deer, or mongoose, they offered us faces that were filled with excited bewilderment. They claimed that unusual people were spotted along the beaches, and with them were floating vessels that were so big they could hold one thousand canoes. We sent a convoy of men to meet with the strangers and find out where they were from and what it was they intended to do. When these men returned, later on, they brought back unusual items – things that piqued our imaginations. The men could not tell us the purpose of these items but said that they were given to them by the foreigners. In exchange, the men offered them whatever that they had with them.

These men offered friendship initially. I met with the leader of this foreign crew myself, and he respectfully offered his hand to me in friendship. He spoke in what seemed like kind words of an unfamiliar language, but we did our best to communicate. It seems that he had been here longer than a few days because some of the people with him were also indigenous to this land. They were people we did not interact with much, however due to their frequent migrations as hunters of the great buffalo.

Some of these men tried to help us understand the foreigner; they told us in hand signs and some words that they were from a distant land where a woman named Queen Isabella reigned. She had sent these men looking for something to bring back to her kingdom. They came to find it and wanted to secure our help. They were fascinated by the many rings of precious metal we wore on our ankles, ears, and wrists, and they inquired with great excitement about where we secured this "gold." They wanted us to show them where we found it. They offered us spicy drinks, clothing, blankets, and several items that we expressed interest in because their color and shape were unusual and fascinating.

After we showed them where to obtain some of the gold they sought, they begged to come to stay with us for shelter and food until one of their other vessels returned with Columbus after a few days. We accommodated the men, but my council of elders was weary. They felt evil spirits in and around them. I even noticed that these men behaved very aggressively. Their hostility towards us grew stronger after just a few days of Columbus leaving for his excursion. They became anxious and bored. Everything took a turn for the worse, however, on the day, one of these men touched one of our innocent ones. This behavior was not our way, and the violence with which he violated this young girl was beyond the realm of anything our people considered acceptable. Infuriated, the great warrior and Chief confronted the man accused and attempted to mete out justice. For his crime, he would be stripped of his belongings, banished, and lose his right hand to the ax of the father whose child he violated - a punishment deemed right and just by the elders.

In response, he spat in the face of the warrior while uttering harsh words in his strange language. Things quickly got out of control as others of his kind came to fight for him. We ordered all 204 of their men out of the village! When they refused to go, a great scuffle ensued, but they eventually retreated into the woods that surrounded the sacred grounds in which we lived and worshiped.

Despite our efforts to ensure they would not return, within a day Columbus and several more hundreds of his men forced their way into my native settlements, brutally slaughtering anyone that came in their way. I could not comprehend the brute force I had allowed on my land. Their violence swallowed small children, older men, and pregnant women alike. The pathways of my once beautiful land ran red with the blood of the Taino people. They hacked the people into pieces, unmercifully slicing open their bellies with their swords. The people of my land were nothing more to them than sheep to be herded viciously to slaughter.

We could not recover from the attack because it happened at night. It was the beginning of our terror, a sign of things more horrific to come. It was like a dark cloud had engulfed our land and the Taino people were like game for slaughter. Christopher Columbus and his crew even laid wagers on whether they could manage to slice a man in two at a stroke, or cut a head from its body, or even disembowel a person with a single blow of the ax.

It pains me to narrate the horrific details of the crimes committed against the helpless and blameless infants of our promised generations. They were violently ripped from their mother's breast only to receive a fate no mother could imagine happening to her child. It is this day that your people celebrate as Columbus day that my people mark as an omen. This historical period in history is forever marked by the brutal red stain of blood.

-King Guacanagari

Divine Intention | Wicked Intention

Now that you have read four powerful stories, my beloved children, I believe your mind should be in deep thought about the meaning behind the actions and behaviors expressed by the characters you just read about. Each story represents one of the four aspects of intention or rather, the four attributions of intent. They are in sequential order based on the stories you've read as follows:

- Clean Face | Pure Heart: an expression of divine intention.
- Clean Face | Impure Heart: an expression of wicked intention.
- Unclean Face | Pure Heart: another expression of divine intention.
- Unclean Face | Impure Heart: another expression of wicked intention.

Allow me to first explain what I mean by *Face, Heart, Clean, Unclean, Pure,* and *Impure* so that you can better understand the allegorical meaning of these terms of art.

Face

Face is a simple term, but with a meaning deeper than you think. Grandchildren, perhaps you have heard the expression *"save face"*? It has a significant meaning that highlights *"to do something that enables people to respect you or to preserve your reputation."*

Saving face is an indication that a person's public persona could be jeopardized or compromised if something is not done otherwise to save it. In simpler terms, my children, if you ever find yourself at a point where you have made a mistake that people around you look down upon – that is when you may find it necessary to take remedial steps to save face. These steps are meant to prevent others from passing unfavorable judgment.

I raise this point because it is instructive. It will help you comprehend that the term of art, *"face,"* is used to explain the attribution of either wicked or divine intent. Keep these ideas in mind moving forward.

Think of *face*, therefore, as being a persona, the way people tend to think of themselves or, better, *how* they hope to be *perceived* by others. *Face*, therefore, indicates the attribution of intent that deals with the *external*, or a mere *perception* of reality that helps us draw conclusions - whether true or false - based on how someone *appears* to us. This is so pervasive in society that a professional mentor might advise you to *dress* for the job you want to acquire, *not* for the one you currently hold.

Imagine that the person on the receiving end of this message is currently a part-time cashier at a local grocery store or fast-food establishment. They might dress in jeans, sneakers, and light collarless t-shirts on a summer workday. Secretly, however, they might aspire to earn a clerkship with a federal judge. Do you think that it would be perceived well by a judge if the potential applicant was first introduced to him or her in this type of casual attire? I don't think so. My experience with judges at the state and federal levels informs my opinion. For the sake of a simpler explanation, *face* is the motivation behind the extra efforts that people put into their appearance when dressing up for church or getting ready for a wedding. This is because they aim to present the best versions of themselves and make a positive, if not lasting, impression on all those in attendance with their appearance.

Right or wrong, people make judgments about others based on what they see. Our perceptions, rooted in the personal beliefs, attitudes, upbringing, and experiences we've had, form the basis for these judgments. There is a very thin line between what is considered constructive criticism and what can be considered an unwarranted judgment. For example, if your boss asks you to *dress* more formally for a meeting with high-profile clients, it sheds light on the level of *professionalism* that is expected at your place of work. However, a comment on your color, weight, features or anything that you *cannot change* about yourself is completely out of the question. So, as your grandmother, I'm telling you to never remain in the company of those who make you feel bad about the way you were born - because whether you like it or not, there will always be people who will try to make it hard for you.

The honorable Dr. King, who was keenly aware of this, thus said that a man should be judged based on the content of his character, not the color of his skin. He said this because America had become a society where justice and injustice were meted out through a caste system based entirely on the dynamic of race. A racial hierarchy structured so that being classified as 'white' inherently meant enjoying all the protections of US citizenship and being a highly melanated person or of African descent meant the denial of citizenship; or not having equal access to the same economic, legal, and political resources given to others. More importantly, it meant the denial of the constitutional protection of due process.

In a racial caste system, *face* becomes even more problematic for the under caste. It further skews the presumption of one character. My beloved children, as you've been reading this book, you already know that there is no shortage of examples when it comes to unequal treatment of our ancestors on the basis of their race. For instance, in the early 1800s, when slavery was legal, a well-dressed black person might be misconstrued as being the property of a thoughtful, wealthy plantation owner who took good care of this *slave*, as opposed to a free, enterprising *businessman* who owns a cotton factory.

In this way, groups are categorically pre-judged to have certain undesirable traits or characteristics. The lower caste was presumed to be either a human chattel, run-away, or thief, while the upper caste was altogether deemed a presumptively good, trustworthy, upright, group of citizens, who were worthy of respect, and given the benefit of the doubt. In a racial caste - like this one, *face* only works to further advantage the dominant or prevailing class by placing them in the upper echelon of society economically, socially, and politically.

In this kind of system, the laws are codified to systematically perpetuate wealth imbalance, produce societal inequities, and ensure that injustice reigns supreme. Eventually, this evolved into an asymmetrical distribution of wealth and power in the nation that effectively placed significant hardships on the achievement of political independence and attainment of generational wealth and prosperity for African people and their descendants.

The key here is to understand that in any society, *face* is a tool. But for people who find themselves situated in a world based on the racial caste system, it represents more than the initial impression. Those who have historically been at the bottom of this racial caste hierarchy, bear a special burden. Their *face* must be carefully curated to avoid the negative stigma associated with their unequal past.

In essence, it means having to care deeply about what people think of you. Thus, a host of expressions meant to admonish the youth about the importance of *face* have been shared over the decades. Some of the many common expressions that speak to this reality include:

- *You never get a second chance to make a first impression*
- *Clothes make the man (or woman)*
- *Dress for the job you want, not the one you have*
- *Never let them see you sweat*
- *You look like a million bucks*
- *Dress how you want to be addressed*

These expressions speak to that aspect of *face*, which alludes to the idea that people are, or at least should be concerned about how they are perceived by others. Imagine seeing a man running toward you with something shaped like a gun in his hand; how you respond to the situation depends on how you feel at that moment. A lot of what you feel in that situation might be driven by how the man *looks,* including his attire. Yes, the way he is dressed plays a huge role in the quick assessment you will make about his *face,* but it also depends on other factors, like the environment in which the event takes place.

For instance, you might feel frightened or insecure if the man running toward you was wearing a mask that completely covered his face, especially if you found yourself located in the midst of a bank robbery. This is in part due to your instincts but also because everything you likely know about the world is based on news reports, crime movies, and your own intelligence which tells you that you should not feel safe. In a split second, you may conclude that he is dangerous and is likely to cause you and others nearby great harm.

Conversely, imagine that the man running towards you in the exact same bank scenario was wearing a militaristic style uniform. How would you feel then? I suspect you might feel a sense of relief that you are going to be saved. You likely drew these conclusions about the intentions of the man running towards you in an instant. All of your decisions were based on the concept of *face.*

Even though we draw a conclusion about the intent of someone based on *face* in an instant as a means of survival, the factors that shape our understanding of appearance or our assessment of people were developed over many years and even generations. Education, movies, individual experiences, social norms, and subconscious behaviors and attitudes help to shape the thinking patterns we engage in daily to prejudge people and objects in our environment.

The person who sees a military uniform might be inclined to think in terms of safety because of any number of factors, including what they learned through their formal education. They may also be inclined to do so because of personal connections to the armed forces through family, a sense of patriotism, or even attitudes formed through media and entertainment. But these responses are relative. Imagine if you were born in a war-torn country and the military was oppressive and violent? Do you think that a person who had this type of experience would associate the uniform with *"safety?"*

It is important to remember this. *Face* can be informative, but It can also be deceiving. If I am successful in my endeavor to impart this important concept, you will learn to use your own *face* strategically, engage with it intelligently in others; and more importantly, you will learn to manage all forms of it cautiously.

These are the kinds of decisions we will make about people, places, and objects every day based on the concept of *face*. This is done in a matter of seconds. Some consider it as prejudging, forming an opinion, or estimation of someone or something *before* applying a careful consideration based on facts. In this day and age, we all do it as a matter of survival.

Heart

At the opposite end of the spectrum, you may hear expressions like *"don't judge a book by its cover,"* *"appearances are misleading,"* *"wolves in sheep's clothes,"* and, *"looks can be deceiving."* These expressions suggest that appearance alone is a poor indicator of who a person really is or what agenda they may have. It also suggests that misjudging someone based on their looks is usually the result of misjudging someone based on *face*.

My grandchildren, have you ever noticed how some people naturally evoke feelings of power, authority, and respect just by walking in the room? They are the kind of people who have an advantageous command over *face*, whether by skill or some inherent gift. Others, on the other hand, find themselves having to work harder just to receive one-third of the respect given to these inherent commanders of *face*. What I mean to say here is that the heart of an individual can actually contradict their persona. Or at least contradict our preconceived notions about their *face* or persona. *I hope that makes sense, beloved grandchildren.*

Think about *heart* as a concept. In fact, it is a little bit easier to explain than *face*, which is something you assign a value to based on appearance alone. *Face*, in the context in which I am speaking about it, does not require proof before a conclusion is drawn. In an instant, we judge whether one is trustworthy and kind or lacking integrity and dangerous.

But listen carefully, grandchildren, because the inverse is true for the attribution of *heart*, which, unlike *face*, resides in the *unseen*. You have to experience *heart* in order to understand it. This is due to the fact that the primary characteristic of *heart* is its invisibility. Therefore, it requires at least some duration of time to analyze, no matter how short or long that period of time might be.

Time, therefore, is another important distinction that helps understand the differences between *face* and *heart*. The relationship between time and *face* is instant. People will size someone up in just a few seconds simply by looking at them. *Heart* is the opposite; you must actually spend time engaging with someone to know what they are really capable of and exactly *what* they intend to do.

In other words, you must actually spend quality time getting to know a person to determine if their outward appearance reflects the truth of their being. Employers, for instance, have a three-month probationary period before they actually roll out all the benefits of full employment for new hires. Do you know why? This evaluation period allows them to assess *heart*. In other words, time answers the important question of whether the person they hired actually reflects the person whose resume initially attracted them and whose stellar interview persuaded them to take a chance on them for the position the company sought to fill.

Employers hire the applicants that appear to be suited or most qualified for the job. If they don't have any direct experience with the applicant (*such as an intern or apprentice*), they must rely on the principle of *face* in making this initial determination. They look at the applicant's resume (*paper*). They reflect on things the applicant said and how well they presented in the interview (*audible and physical impressions*). They assess the applicants' stated hobbies and activities to see if they are well-rounded (*personal life*). And they research the applicant's occupational skills with references (*professional development*). But the true test of character comes from hiring the new employee and placing them on probation for a period of time (*usually three months*) if the employee maintains *face* or proves their ability on the job while showing that they are coachable and a team player, in most cases, the employer will extend the full benefits of the company permanently.

Time is one of the most effective ways to assess *heart* attribution. Another important observation to note about *heart* is that it is often spoken of in terms of its locality.

To illustrate, let's look at some common expressions you may have used or heard that relate to *heart*:

- *Let's get down to the heart of the matter*
- *She wears her heart on her sleeve*

Both of these statements interestingly point to a location. *Did you notice grandchildren?* The first expression suggests that *heart* is not located up high where it might be easy to access. In this way try to imagine that *heart* is like a particular piece of clothing hiding at the very bottom of a full laundry basket. It has to be searched for underneath layers of concealment. One might notice an unusual smell coming from a source in or near the laundry room. They may dig through the basket of dirty clothes until they realize that the unpleasant smell was a pair of mildewy beach shorts!

The second expression also suggests locality; here, the *heart* is worn on the sleeve, meaning the way this person is on the inside betrays her by showing up through her emotional behavior in spite of the outward expressions she wears or her *face*. In other words, she may be dressed like a fierce, confident boss, but her behavior quickly reveals insecurity. In truth, she may be someone who is really easy to manipulate and might even be a poor manager. A timid nature and desire to avoid confrontation at all costs reveal the *heart* of this woman, and her employees, who have witnessed her cower in the face of minor disputes, show a lack of respect towards her for this apparent lack of authority.

Clean | Unclean

The words "*clean*" and "*unclean*" are a very common part of the English Language. One can say that something *clean* could mean something that is *sanitary*, but understanding the complex language we speak requires context above anything else. My grandchildren, what I am shedding light on here is the fact that sometimes "*clean* and *unclean*" goes beyond their surface meaning. Sometimes, you have to dig deeper where the words "*clean*" and "*unclean*" are concerned. They could highlight the willingness found in our intentions to fit into our respective communities and play the role we have been given in our lives.

You might follow a pattern; wear a uniform; and represent yourself in a way that people expect you to represent yourself. Therefore, *"clean"* is a term of art in this context that means *acceptable to our sense of normalcy.* Think about the expression, *"that guy cleaned up well,"* or *"he was clean as a whistle."* Both of these expressions mean that somehow a person's physical appearance has transformed into something that is acceptable to the standards set by the beholder.

This, in fact, happened to me once. Let me tell you what happened...

During law school, I wore my hair in a big voluminous puff that was gathered neatly on the top of my head. It looked like a high bun. My professor admonished me to *"clean up"* and do a more *traditional* look for my interview with the large law firm where I hoped to do a summer clerkship. *Reluctantly*, I straightened my hair. I would not advise doing this. However, I was facing severe financial hardship at the time and everything in my life was at stake. My hope was that straight hair would help me eliminate any excuses that the firm might use to deny me the opportunity based on their perception of *face*.

When I reported to the professor, after what seemed to be a successful interview with Gardere Wynn Sewell, LLP., she looked me up and down before exclaiming proudly, *"You cleaned up well!"* What she meant by that statement was that I had met *her* expectations and standards for what an African American attorney should look like when representing the law school.

When I say *"unclean"* again in this book, it is a term of art. It does not mean that I looked *"dirty"* or *"ill-groomed"* to her, but I just simply did not meet *her* standards in my natural state. Therefore, *"unclean"* means *unacceptable* to our cultural, societal, and spiritual norms. Both *"clean"* and *"unclean"* are terms of art that apply to *face* attributions, meaning someone on their appearance gives us the sense that they are willing and able to live up to our expectations. These expectations can be based on societal norms or on one's ability to appear within the molds we've established for them based on our social rules or religious constructs.

Pure | Impure

Pure is another term of art. It means the person's behavior is in alignment with their *face* or how they present themselves physically based on the sense of sight, hearing, and touch. It alludes to the idea that a person is being *transparent* about what they intend to do. They don't operate in ways that contradict themselves in fact or theory. If someone's behavior, in turn, doesn't align with what they say they are about, then this is considered to fall under the *impure* attribution.

I want you to know this, my beloved ones; what I am telling you is one of those things about life I want you to be *keenly* aware of. I am speaking as a matter of fact, not judgment. I want you to be cognizant of this aspect of the human condition because it has been the way things have been done for millennia. *Face & heart* are the terms of art I have used to teach you this important knowledge. I do so in order for you to learn, teach, and conduct yourselves effectively and with wisdom. I was not taught this information. I had to acquire it through self-observation, acuity of insight, and through observations made while engaging with society in various capacities. Having this knowledge might not seem all that great right now, but I promise you it will come in handy in the future.

My children, remember Julissa? Can you imagine if Julissa had been aware of *clean face | impure heart* prior to meeting Michael? How different would her life be? Julissa grossly misunderstood Michael's ambitions, character, and intentions. Although Michael seemed like a friend with his big, toothy smile, soothing voice, charm, and gentle disposition, Julissa would not have been so forthcoming to him about her personal family life if she had knowledge of this concept. She would have known to be more cautious in the presence of someone who seemed only to be a person of *clean face*. She would have waited a year and possibly longer to observe his true intentions and character while gauging the depth and scope of his business ambitions.

Michael displayed a classic case of *clean face | impure heart*. By presenting himself as a confidant and a colleague, he induced Julissa to let her guard all the way down. He looked, talked, and presented himself in ways that Julissa found consistent with *normal* behavior - or ways acceptable to her standards. She trusted him right off. She assumed, based on her assessments about his *face* or outward appearance, that he cared about her. She thought he had her best interest at *heart*.

I want to note here that *face* can be upheld over an extended period of time. Sometimes just long enough to earn someone's trust without question. We have all been guilty of extending someone the benefit of the doubt without having any reliable data or justification for doing so. Unfortunately for Julissa, she had to learn this lesson about *clean face | impure heart* the hard way.

Now, my children, let's talk about how similarly King Guacanagari and his people suffered a deadly fate due to his inability to assess Christopher Columbus, who represented the attribution, unclean *face | impure heart*. Why was Columbus' *face unclean*? Let me remind you of the meaning of *unclean* as a term of art. Here it means something *"outside the realm of normalcy for the behaviors, customs, and beliefs of a particular society."* King Guacanagari should have been on high alert simply because he was engaging with someone who was alien to his culture, customs, traditions and ways of life.

This does not mean to say that we should automatically assume that differences are dangerous, but we should not automatically assume something new, unfamiliar, and unrecognizable is safe either. The two are not the same. I hope you understand what I'm trying to convey to you, my children, because time and again, history has proven my point.

On a pleasant note, *clean face | pure heart* is represented in the story of Grandmother Betty's character and her conduct with Mr. Cecil and the management of his resources. Mr. Cecil was completely dependent on my grandmother for her accurate and honest relay of how much income he earned daily. Without this information, he could not effectively pay his bills, buy groceries, support his weekly assistance, and live functionally. *Clean face* was my grandmother's outward appearance to a man with no eyes. He relied on the sound of her voice, the touch of her hands, and the comfort of her spirit in order to determine whether or not she was indeed his trusted confidant.

Mr. Cecil was not unwise; he had other ways of verifying information provided to him by my grandmother. For instance, Mr. Cecil often had someone else he knew and trusted to count the money prior to my grandmother when possible. He also had other methods of testing Grandmother Betty's honesty. But time after time, she proved herself true to serving his best interest, and they remained in a close relationship with one another and grounded in trust.

Now, my precious grandchildren, the best story of all to me was the example of *unclean face | pure heart* with the diamond ring as the vehicle for assessing its nature from several angles. First, the homeless man represents *unclean face* but not for the reasons you might be thinking. *Unclean,* here is a term of art that simply indicates unacceptable standards based on societal, personal, or behavioral norms. His condition as a homeless person makes him appear to the rest of the world as someone out of the realm of normalcy. He is not, by most accounts, considered to be an upright citizen capable of contributing or playing a beneficial role in society.

That is what *unclean* means in this context. However, he proved what we all need to be mindful of when interacting with individuals. That is, never judge a person by *face* alone. And as you can clearly see based on the outcome of this story, the man possessed a physical *"heart"* of gold, and his heart attribution was as transparent as a diamond.

Chapter 6

Sacred Wellness

Head | Womb | Feet

When I was young, it seemed like Grandmother Betty was always making a fuss over three distinct areas of my body. In fact, at one point, I thought she was obsessed with my feet, my womb, and my head.

Girls around the world are celebrated when their bodies begin to menstruate. For example, in South Africa, when a girl has her first period, the family celebrates the event with a special party. Female guests, family, and friends join in to shower the girl with blessings and gifts and to wish her a long, healthy, and fertile life. Men are forbidden to see her during the event.

What's important here to understand is that more than the period, it is the emphasis on fertility that brings attention to women in this regard. But *why*? Well, my beautiful grandchildren, this is the Divine Path laid out for women. As women, our bodies are designed to create life – something that the opposite sex cannot do, even if they tried. At the same time, our body becomes more than just a collection of parts because our womb has a sacred responsibility. A responsibility to carry on a race.

All of this made much more sense to me as I grew and began to understand why my Grandmother was always so concerned.

Let me tell you a little something about how my Grandmother took care of me in the days of my youth. I can't help but smile every time I think about her voice, her advice, and her knowledge about Divine Health and Wellness, specifically about our feet, womb, and head.

I can remember as if it were only yesterday how she was always concerned about my foot health and constantly admonished me to elevate my feet for 15 to 20 minutes at the end of each day. She said this was important for my blood and my health.

She would also narrate how back in those days, she and her mother, Great-grandmother Lena Mae, worked as cleaning ladies in hotels for some time. They were always standing on their feet, so both she, and Great-grandmother Lena Mae were sure to spend some time elevating their feet above their heads. Elevating their legs at a 45 degree angle over the heart for about 25 minutes gave them ample time to relax and feel good after a tiring day.

Not only was this a great way to relax, but it was also an act that came with several medical benefits! As a result of her practices, my grandmothers had beautiful, shapely legs, and they never had vein problems. My Grandmother Betty attributed this to the attention they gave to the legs by propping them up on three or four pillows to be on a certain angle enabling a direct blood flow towards the head after hours of standing.

Another thing I remember when I was really young was how my Grandmother insisted on having my feet soaked in bubbly water with salts and special oils. The bubbly water always filled the **air** with the aroma of sweet mints intertwined with something earthy that I don't exactly remember. This, she said, was to ensure that I had healthy, soft, sturdy feet. I distinctly remember the blue tub with an extension cord that she plugged into the wall before pressing a button that made the bubbles rise in the water warm. This type of water therapy was a part of my childhood experiences and early training in the many aspects of *Divine SelfQare*.

I also avoid placing my feet directly on cold hard floor surfaces. This is also one of the reasons why hard flat sandals are bad for your feet because they can never be in harmony with the natural curves of your feet. These practices are part of my daily routine to this day. Whether it's a foot massage or a foot soak, taking care of your feet is essential – after all, they are what carry us through life.

All the things that I have highlighted above have been my Grandmother Betty's greatest admonishment to me. As soon as I rose from a bed or chair to walk, my Grandmother could hear me and would yell, *"Sheila, don't walk around without your house slides! You'll get arthritis when you're old."* Many folk from her generation believed and taught that the source of arthritis was from years of cold entering the bones through the bottoms of your feet. This also included walking over concrete tiles or other cold but unsafe indoor flooring. It was a definite no in her presence. Therefore, when it comes to the health of your feet, warmth is key! Even today, I adhere to this practice. However, today I mostly enjoy walking barefoot on carpeted floors that I get cleaned annually by professional carpet sanitation companies.

If clean and healthy feet were essential to my Grandmother, then a clean and healthy *womb* was like a sacred religious custom or practice. No area brought me more anxiety in my youth around my Grandmother than the day of the month when my cycle started. Not only was I forbidden to sit in a body of water to bathe, but I also had to have a special pot for cleaning that area of my body. Disposing of the sanitary napkins was more than cumbersome because I had to tightly seal the napkin and conceal it in a paper or plastic bag that wouldn't betray its hidden contents before walking down the hall to the incinerator for what I called a 'proper burial.'

To my Grandmother, this act was necessary for the maintenance of hygiene *and* spiritual protection. Cleanliness was not only next to godliness; it *was* godliness. In my Grandmother's mind, a woman's menses or menstrual blood was a dangerous material that exposed women to vulnerability. Any improper handling was tantamount to an invitation to spiritual harm from those who do evil deeds through wicked designs.

Therefore, it was essential to clean myself up properly during my cycle. It was also necessary to completely dispose of my napkins. I can't imagine what lengths Grandmother Betty would have gone to if the incinerator weren't available. It would have taken nothing less than destroying my soiled pads in an actual *fire* to relieve her!

These were things I dared not to question my Grandmother about. I was pretty confident that her adherence was based on actual lessons learned directly from experience. My Grandmother also believed in douching, something that was considered trendy among certain classes of women from her generation.

Douching is an act that requires you to spray or shower your vagina with water or any other cleansing liquids. She douched her private part with a little bit of vinegar and warm water, which helped her keep it fresh. Vinegar was a great addition because it is known to cut odor and also work as an antibacterial. My Grandmother added douching to her regular routine, which helped her to control and maintain her reproductive health, especially after sexual intercourse, childbirth, and menstrual cycles. Even though I have not made douching a part of my *Divine SelfQare Strategy*, I do engage in another form of hydrotherapy related to the vagina. This process is called vaginal steaming – something we will discuss later in this book.

The final most crucial aspect of my body that my Grandmother took particular notice of was my head. As I mentioned before, Grandmother Betty was very concerned about femininity, hygiene practices, and appearance. Still, she was equally worried about the health of my head. Her focus was on having a healthy, clean mouth. She brushed her teeth and gargled with mouthwash twice a day, once in the morning and once before bed. She always advised me to do the same. Other than a fresh and healthy mouth, she was always concerned about having clean, presentable ears and also stressed the importance of not straining my eyes. She also had one other area that she instilled in me to notice. I was to pay attention to the crevices around my nose. This area is known to house a lot of dead skin cells and bacteria. She employed a strategy for removing them with the round end of a hairpin before exfoliating the face with a safe, all-natural facial scrub. Not only did this give me smooth skin, but it also kept any acne or whiteheads from forming.

Grandmother Betty's focus on these body parts always remained with me. However, at the time, I didn't agree with everything she did; I honestly just thought she was old-fashioned and sometimes downright excessive. My children, when we are young, we do not tend to see things as deeply as our parents or grandparents do. In this manner, I didn't fully understand the significance of these special wellness skills and habits. However, as the years went by, life had a way of constantly honing in on the ancient wisdom, traditions, and healing practices of those very wise women who made up the matriarchy of our family. As I write this book, I wish to be the beacon of knowledge for all of my beloved grandchildren.

Grandmother Betty was the last link in the chain for me, and now I am that link for you. Her work was shared with me through stories and action that expressed her desire to see me experience, what I *now* call *Divine Health and Wellness*. These experiences were, in truth, vestiges of an even more beautiful and ancient past where we as African daughters of the Most High enjoyed many therapeutic, beautiful womb, feet, and head wellness and cleansing modalities.

As you read on, I want to shed some light on my sacred awakening. Each one of us, at some point in our lives, comes face to face with a situation that (*almost spiritually*) shows us the path that we have to choose. Similarly, I want to tell you about an interaction I had many years ago that led me on the mission to bestow this Divine Knowledge on all of you.

African Origins of Divine SelfQare | The Awakening

Now, my beloved children, listen closely as I narrate to you an experience that gave my life and my work a whole new meaning.

A few years ago, a Houston spa owner and friend by the name of Aneisha Daneen, convinced me to take her certification program in vaginal steaming. She seemed determined to usher me into this unique field. It was like she knew that one day I would make a special contribution to the world of womb wellness. After finally accepting her offer, I decided to open up and discuss my new business venture with a coworker. To protect her privacy, I'll refer to her by the name Bola Tobi.

Bola is a Nigerian-born attorney who migrated to the US in her 30's. I told Bola about my mobile or in-home vaginal steaming service and inquired as to whether she'd be interested in the experience.

I was intrigued when she turned around abruptly and asked,

"What do you know about vaginal steaming?
My people have been doing that for ages, if not longer!"

I looked at her with the kind of wonder that must accompany the face of a child who recently woke up to discover a dime underneath her pillow just hours after suffering the loss of a tooth.

"Wait, what do you mean, Bola?
African women do vaginal steaming?"

My children, you won't believe how surprised I was when Bola nodded and proceeded to tell me about the practice of vaginal steaming as a healing remedy for new mothers after childbirth.

Interestingly, the story that Bola relayed to me was familiar – it was a saga that plays itself out generationally. One rooted in the conflict between preserving the old ways versus someone with a new mind, adapting to the norms and standards set by the west today. Old and new ways of life often clash when it boils down to matters of health, medicine, and therapy. In this manner, Bola narrated a story that told about both the importance of Divine Wellness in practice and how it has been a traditional custom that has trickled down generationally by way of the elders.

Your grandmother listened with much intent, as Bola talked about how her mother-in-law, Mama Yemi, traveled all the way to the United States from Nigeria to help Bola recover from a long, arduous labor and to welcome the birth of her first grandchild – a beautiful baby girl, born to her very own son and daughter-in-law.

In families around the world, new grandmothers usually take responsibility for caring for their daughter-in-law post-childbirth. They are seen as the perfect individual to take care of the new mother and child because of their aged wealth of knowledge. To honor a similar tradition, Mama Yemi sought to recover Bola after her delivery.

After the hospital released Bola to go home with the baby, Mama Yemi immediately proceeded to prepare a steam-filled bath with special herbs meant to restore Bola's womb to its pre-birth natural condition. Even though Mama Yemi intended for her to begin the treatment by sitting directly over the steam for thirty minutes, Bola had already decided how she wanted her body to heal.

You see, children, here we see how Mama Yemi (*who was a clear believer in Divine Health and Wellness*) tried to do what she thought was right for her daughter-in-law. According to traditional ways of the women from her community, this was something necessary for both sexual health and overall womb healing for women who had recently given birth.

Now, Bola, a woman following the ways of western medicine, chose her own path. This led to an unexpected problem between the two. Mama Yemi did not calculate that Bola would uphold the advice of western doctors over her own. These modern-day doctors had advised Bola not to engage in vaginal steaming after being released from their care over her own healing wisdom and traditions.

The doctors also claimed that if Bola engaged in vaginal steaming, she would destroy the delicate stitching she carries to support the vaginal tears she suffered during childbirth and delivery.

When Bola refused to steam, Mama Yemi became livid, accusing her of prioritizing western medicine over thousands of years' worth of womb wisdom and traditions practiced by the women of her lineage for generations. The two engaged in a heated argument before the mother-in-law admonished her for refusing to steam as she advised her to do. This refusal, she claimed, would result in Bola no longer being any good to her husband.

Bola was firm in her position and determined not to disobey the doctors' orders. She did, however, agree to eat the traditional foods that her mother-in-law prepared. Mama Yemi made several super foods to help Bola's body cleanse and heal on its own. Dishes like pepper and vegetable soups loaded with greens like bitter leaves. She also consumed a special cornmeal porridge designed to aid breast milk production.

It's very important to understand that the conflict here is not between two women. Instead, it's between two schools of thought: ancient wellness versus western medicine.

So, my children, do you think one of the women might be wrong? I wouldn't say so. See, as people who take time to immerse our minds in Divine Knowledge, it is also crucial to learn how to respect other people's opinions.

Bola, an adult, who just went through the miracle of birth had just become a mother. At this point, she has her own perception of what is right for her and her baby. At the same time, Mama Yemi also wanted the best for her daughter-in-law and grandchild, but only harbored a different belief system when it came to wellness and healing.

You see my beloved; it all comes down to **Divine Intent**. Both women held no negatives for each other in their hearts. Even though they disagreed on how Bola should heal, they both wanted the same result. This shows us that both of them had pure intentions. Undoubtedly, when people harbor pure intentions, good things always happen one way or the other.

Eventually, Bola did permit Mama Yemi to help her steam, even though it was after quite some time.

Even though Mama Yemi was not considering the fact that Bola had stitches, it is important to see where she is coming from. Through her seasoned experiences, Mama Yemi was keenly aware that many women before her own daughter-in-law had similar tears that, if given proper time and healing treatment, would also heal naturally due to ancient practices like vaginal steaming.

This story was a revelation to me. All I had heard about vaginal steaming up to this point suggested that it originated from Asian cultures and that it had absolutely no connection to the numerous African cultures that existed for millennia. This was one time when I was glad the information I had been given was wrong!

More importantly, this insight from Bola began my quest for more information about the African origins of vaginal steaming. I also noticed a correlation to some of the very things that my own Grandmother felt strongly about regarding vaginal health. Moreover, it reminded me of the care that women from her era received from other female relatives and members of the community after childbirth, especially when none was available in terms of professional medical assistance or treatment.

I was always curious to learn more about the origins of these ancient practices. In my research and studies, I found that several million African women were abducted from their homelands and brought against their wills to the colonies. Even after being forced to live in foreign lands, many of them still engaged in their traditional practices when and wherever possible. A majority of these practices were related to womb health, childbirth, and reproduction. Many more of these practices endured through the course of slavery and were passed down from generation to generation through midwives and traditional healers. Sacred children, it is because of their endurance that we have the privilege of learning these practices today.

The reason why I termed this my awakening is because I felt naturally determined to learn even more about what the ancestors had to offer. To know what wellness strategies they engaged in for head, womb, and feet care meant opening up to a world of divine possibilities and being vulnerable to the process. I suddenly felt so connected to the rich yet tumultuous history of our people. My search for the truth would take me on a journey in and out of African-owned clothing and hair shops speaking with Senegalese, Nigerian, Ghanaian, Ethiopian, and Gambian women.

My insatiable quest for knowledge proved useful; eventually, landing me much closer to home than I anticipated. My children, this is where I met an Ethiopian sister, by the name of Yeshimebet, a woman who would reveal to me something so astonishing and so rewarding to my heart and mind that the next segment is fully dedicated to her.

In fact, Mama Yeshimebet affirmed what I already knew in my heart and soul. She was proof of the fact that I was heading down a path that was good and right. She was the Divine Affirmation proving all the powerful insights my own Grandmother Betty had been preparing me for my whole life. Today, I sum up all of our matriarchs insights and teachings using this simple term: *Total Body Alignment* through *Divine SelfQare*.

Quest for Truth | Journey in the Aisles

Before I begin this story, I would like to share how lucky I have been to meet such people. From Bola to the people I am about to tell you about, I am thankful to each one of them. Not only did they help me on my quest, but they also strengthened my respect for the ways of my ancestors. Through their words and sayings, I felt like I was exactly where I should have been all along. Their input completed my study in ways that I may not have been able to do myself.

So, if today you find yourself reading these stories, it's because the Most High was most gracious towards your loving grandmother. Alright now, let's begin.

This lovely encounter takes place at a nearby store where your grandmother was shopping for some household basics. Trust me when I say this, I never thought that a trip to a home store would be so enlightening!

One day, I was perusing through the aisles of a popular department store when I ran into a young woman. She lived at the same complex I lived in for the first four years of my return to Maryland. Her name was Selam, and she was a young, beautiful, and outgoing Ethiopian girl. As I glanced at her, it turned out that she remembered me too!

After a quick greeting, we spoke with great interest about each other's lives, especially when I shared my new business endeavor of vaginal steaming with her. Once again, I was astounded when she responded:

"Oh, we do that in Ethiopia too!"

I almost fell out of my seat, but I wasn't sitting down anywhere!. How was this happening? Once again, I had asked for historical data from the Most High to help me learn about the specific practice of vaginal steaming from an African Woman health perspective. And once again, I was getting a clear reply.

Only this time it was echoing from the voice of a babe, leading me closer to my destination. You see my sacred children, the Most High has been with me at every step. It is with divine grace that I was able to receive such enlightening information.

Naturally, I shot her with questions. She said she didn't know the exact name of the practice but that she would send me information describing how it was done in Ethiopia. She explained it in a way that shook me with curiosity:

"They dig this hole in the ground and put a special herb in it... and smoke comes out. And they sit down over it with the special covering that allows the smoke to rise up...
They sweat really hard...
and then they also melt this kind of butter on their head at the same time ...."

What? I couldn't believe my ears. The Ethiopian sisters had been using the most extensive and earthy processes of vaginal smoking – one that seemed to incorporate the same three body parts I had been raised to care for from childhood by my own Grandmother Betty – the head, the womb, and the feet!

Oh, my beloved granddaughters and grandsons, I only wish you had experienced how ecstatic I was when I heard Selam's words. It was an incredible feeling because in my mind I was busy intertwining what she was telling me with the comprehensive teachings of my wise Grandmother. It truly did put things into divine, historical perspective!

Anyway, back to the story!

I was so intrigued when I reached home that I found myself texting her for the information she promised even before I could properly put down my shopping bags. She eventually sent me some links to a couple of YouTube videos a few weeks later. But there was one problem. The people giving the vital info I needed about vaginal smoking were speaking in a dialect of Amharic, an Ethiopian language. I could not speak nor understand what they were saying in Amharic; neither could Selam. But still, she offered another solution. She promised to ask her mom, who went by the name 'Yeshi,' which is short for 'Yeshimebet,' meaning *Queen of Thousands*, if she would translate the video for me.

Months went by, and I inquired frequently, but there was always some reason that prevented her mother from speaking to me. But this small setback did not deter my effort to get the answers I needed. I contacted every Ethiopian woman in Silver Spring that I knew. I even talked to women I didn't know. Women that I encountered at the Ethiopian-owned hair salons and restaurants I patronized in downtown Silver Spring, MD, or elsewhere within the DMV.

Still, there was never a sufficient answer, and many times I felt like I was being ignored or dismissed. It was frustrating because I knew this information was somehow connected to a vital fulfillment of my *Divine Purpose* in life. At least, I was beginning to draw the right parallels between the concept of

Total Body Alignment and the ancient modalities of sacred *African healing* and wellness traditions.

The way I saw it, African women had been delivering babies from the earliest point of human history. As the mothers of civilizations, there was no way that African women had not made significant contributions to womb health and wellness practices like vaginal steaming that were both holistic and enduring. I knew I was right on the brink of something special and could tell by the sensation running through my bones.

Now comes a very interesting turn in my story. Since I was not having much luck getting answers from my beautiful but protective Ethiopian sisters, one day I tried my luck with an Ethiopian brother instead!

I saw him selling his amazing, new Injera chips and lentil dip products at a local grocery store in my area. After tasting some of his samples, I proceeded with, *"may I ask you a question about vaginal health practices of Ethiopian women?"* He seemed slightly taken aback at first, but the respectful and inquisitive tone of my voice probably allowed him to see that I was coming from the perspective of a student and a sincere researcher.

I explained to him that I had recently learned about a form of vaginal steaming, or rather smoking, among Ethiopian women. However, I still needed answers to some of my pressing questions like:

What was it called?

What did the women burn in the hole to create the smoke?

And more importantly, what was the proper name for "vagina" and/or "womb" in Amharic, the main language spoken by many Ethiopians?

The man looked to be middle-aged, but he had been in the US for many years, so thankfully, he was not offended by my questions. To my surprise, he answered them rather helpfully, at least whatever ones he could, and I left the encounter with just a little more knowledge and insight. I also understood why it had been so difficult to acquire answers to my questions. He explained to me that for Ethiopian women, such topics were *not easy* to discuss.

This raised another important question in my mind. So, I asked him, *"How then would an Ethiopian woman relay her reproductive health concerns or needs to her doctor?"* He explained that typically, an Ethiopian woman would simply refer to her vagina indirectly as 'woman parts,' likely by using a common metaphor. He further tried to pronounce and explain that the actual word for a vagina in Amharic as *"mmmphs"* or *"emese."* But *"emese"* was typically not uttered out loud.

In several cultures today, women are not given the freedom to talk about their bodies. Those who choose to have open conversations about their vaginas, menstrual cycles, or reproductive health are usually looked down upon. Women are oftentimes expected to remain silent on such important topics – all in the name of modesty. Thankfully, the man I met was more than willing to continue the conversation with me despite his hesitant demeanor.

I asked him to clarify whether *"emese"* was equivalent to the brash English word *"P-U-S"*. I felt I should just spell out the first three letters instead of the whole word. Leaving the last two letters out made the word seem less jarring. Plus, I hoped it would avoid making an already awkward conversation – while in the middle of a grocery store aisle filled with consumers - even more difficult to pursue.

The outcome of my brief encounter with this Ethiopian man was very generous but not complete. However, I took away essential concepts from this experience, but nothing as exciting or powerful as I'd soon learn about from a very special source.

As we move on to the final part of the story, I want to tell you how effort and hard work is almost always the key to achieving something great. After my awakening, I did not ever stop myself from exploring. It is because of my zeal and child-like quest for knowledge that I was able to compile this book that you are reading today.

Everything I gathered up to this point had been instrumental on the journey that set me on this very course. I chose to develop my teachings about the *Divine SelfQare Strategy* so that my children and grandchildren could arm themselves with this significant knowledge. One day during an extended period of fasting and prayer, I received an unexpected text on my cell phone. It was a message that finally presented me with the answer to a question I had been asking for months, *"What more do I have to learn from my Ethiopian sisters?"* The person who sent me the text was Selam, the young Ethiopian girl I ran into a few months back while shopping in College Park for one of my new client's custom-designed at-home spas. She indicated that her mother, who was familiar with the traditional vaginal wellness practices used by some Ethiopian women, was ready and willing to talk with me. I dialed her right away!

Queen Of Thousands | Yeshimebet Speaks

After exchanging warm greetings with her, I explained to Yeshimebet that I was researching the role of African women in developing holistic health and womb wellness strategies, particularly vaginal steaming or smoking. This sparked a two-hour-long conversation that left me feeling so inspired that I literally could not talk about the conversation to anyone for weeks. My head was reeling. I learned so many vital concepts and received answers to so many questions that I felt obligated to tell her how grateful I was for opening up to me and sharing this sacred wisdom simply because I asked.

We discussed ancient practices like vaginal smoking. I took so many notes because the new words, expressions, and metaphors she taught me were so beautiful and innocent-sounding to my ears that tears swelled in my eyes, and I began to cry. I felt like I had a spiritually enlightening experience, an awakening of the feminine essence as engaged in for generations by our ancestors. I felt like I was being let in on something sacred, a secret that once belonged to me - and being mine, I had a duty to regain what was somehow sadly lost many centuries ago.

This collective wisdom and knowledge belonging to African women spoke about our wombs in such precious, rhythmic, and sacred tones. It was almost unbelievable to think that this sacred aspect of womanhood could be expressed with such eloquence and prose as in the Amharic word, "*Dabo,*" meaning "*beautiful bread.*" My beloved, can you imagine such a sweet form of expression being used between lovers? Or see how such an endearing term could be used to introduce adolescent girls to their feminine essence? Such soft and gentle phrases are a stark contrast to the vulgar terms used by men and women in popular culture to express the parts of the female reproductive system today. It is almost shameful to see how such a sacred part of a woman's body is reduced to such words. These terms deprive us of a deep sense of personal value and sacred intimacy and, unfortunately, put the bodies of women on public display much like a carton of cheap eggs are put out front because they are about to spoil in the next 24 hours.

Social media constantly floods our electronic device screens with nudity and soft pornography, masquerading itself as creative expressions of art, music, and dance. I can't help but feel the deep sense of shame and disappointment the spirits of our great matriarchs might be feeling in some capacity today. Whether as a mother, grandmother, or even an aunt, no matriarch wants to see her flesh and blood be shamed or demeaned on the basis of her womanhood.

Did they struggle, die, or risk their lives and personal well-being just to have the minds of their descendants groomed toward a life of licentiousness masquerading as a distorted type of women's liberation movement? My beautiful grandchildren, most people unintentionally show just how disconnected they are from the hopes and dreams of our noble ancestors. Understand the feminine essence of women like Fannie Lou Hamer, Ida B. Wells, Coretta Scott King, Betty Shabazz, Amy Jacques Garvey, Hazel Scott, and Maggie Lena Walker. These women could never have imagined a world where young children are introduced to musical lyrics that brag about crime and sexual exploits. Perhaps, what's worse is how today's performer encourages everyone else to dance to debauchery and sheer exploitation.

Truth be told, these realities trouble my soul so much they have become a part of the motivations I have for writing this book. To protest this debauchery on behalf of our elders and my beloved granddaughters, on your behalf as well. You descend from noble women - *from royalty* - you should know this. You should seek to perpetuate the honor and legacy of our family's matriarchs *and* our collective ancestors. QM Harriet Tubman and QM Jacobs lived honorable lives in spite of their circumstances. You should aspire to do the same.

To me, any knowledge and education worthy of being passed down from one generation about womanhood must include these elders. My goal with this book is to achieve this very thing. If all goes accordingly, I might even set my heart on creating another book dedicated to the legacy of our honor-worthy matriarchs. I would title it, *The 19 Matriarchs*. Not only would it be an expression and labor of love, but it would also be a way for me to pay them my respects while giving their knowledge and teachings a vehicle to reach you, sacred grandchildren.

One of the reasons I'd pursue writing such a book is to defend the legacy of our ancestors, who would have never imagined that their sacred daughters, the promised *heirs* of their *hopes* and dreams, would be willing to *self-identify* as a euphemism for a four-legged animal, prostitute, witch, or 'whore.' These words once were hurled to diminish the value and dignity of our ancestors' humanity. And it is imperative that you know, they fought tooth and nail to be free of these indignities.

Today, you will find two kinds of artists in the music industry. One that actually respects the craft and the other kind who would have you believe that these indignities and exploitations are actually modern badges of honor because they are *self-inflicted*. What they won't tell you is how they have sold their souls for money and along with their souls went their self-respect.

It is sad to see how most modern-day artists have forgotten what music is supposed to be about. It no longer appears to be a pick-me-up tune; instead, it's three minutes of cussing and references to immodesty or sex here and there. What I mean to convey here, beloved, is that music has the power to make people feel and express things that perhaps a plain conversation can't. Why waste that precious platform on such vulgar and carnal things?

Many people in the industry operate in a vacuum of pure individualism. They neither care about nor research the works of those who came before them in the spirit of collective progress using **Sankofa**. So, what do they care if these derogatory terms, so commonly used today, go much deeper into history? But they *should* care. These words were derived from the horrific exploitations and rape of women and little girls who were torn away from their families and forced to endure chattel slavery. The kind of terms meant to demoralize them as unworthy Jezebels, lowly dogs, and sometimes, to even demonize them with accusations of *witchcraft*. Perhaps, these atrocious terms became nothing more than a self-serving means of deflecting the immoral behavior of those enslavers who oppressed them.

Therefore, when an artist uses these terms they are merely perpetuating the behaviors of former slave holders, the same oppressors who raped, demeaned, and demoralized our ancestors.

Music artists and performers should align their talents with positive messages that uplift people, so that when their music reaches the corners of the globe, it represents harmony, love, and most of all – inspires us to respect one another, honoring our humanity and gender.

Now, you might be asking, *how did we end up here*? Well, my beloved granddaughters and grandsons, as simple as that question is, the answer is complicated. But one thing is for sure; it has much to do with a great disconnect or break in the chain that links the hopes, values, and aspirations of one generation to its successive generations.

That being said, all of this brings me to realize how this book is so important to you, my beloved granddaughters and sons. Even though I may be long assigned to the kingdom of heaven by the time you access this writing, you have no excuse or justification for neglecting the divine ways of healing and wisdom traditions as realized here in this book and taught by our ancestors.

You know who you are. You know what your Divine Purpose is connected to. You know how to access and fulfill your sacred duty as a human to perpetuate Divine Health and Wellness through *Divine SelfQare*. Moreover, you should never forget that the Most High has given you everything you need to be virtuous, independent, victorious, and fearless – the sacred and essential tools of **Air, Fire, Earth,** and **Water** that when coupled with **Divine Intent**, create those *trans-physical* weapons the Most High ordained for you as ambassadors of Divine Health and facilitators of *Divine SelfQare*.

Chapter 7

Denkenesh

My beloved children, when I was young, I found stories that my grandmother told me incredibly fascinating, mostly because they were always filled with wonder, mystique, and most importantly, a life lesson that I could store in my heart forever.

In this manner, I wish to tell you stories and anecdotes that can help you resonate with the characters so that you can grasp the *Divine Knowledge* and concepts that I have wanted to highlight in this book.

Through the eyes of a special woman, who lived a long time ago in Ethiopia, I want you to experience the origins of the *Divine SelfQare Strategy* and how women before us embraced Divine Healing practices that still continue to serve us today.

Now, let's meet Denkenesh and discover a sacred way of wellness through a day in her life...

It was a warm, sunny day in *Raya*, a small village where Denkenesh lived with her husband, Bereket, and their two young sons, Michael and Samson. Looking through the window of her living quarters, Denkenesh observed her husband working diligently to put the final touches on the *"Gojo"* or *cottage* that he built for her to engage in the ancient way of wellness. For Bereket to take up such an endeavor on behalf of the woman he cherished was a gesture of love. His feelings for Denkenesh were deeply rooted in family values and friendship. It is true. Denkenesh was not just a wife to Bereket. She was his best friend. He loved her with his whole heart and would go to great lengths to make her happy.

The reasons Bereket adored his wife were many. But the fact that she bore him two healthy, rambunctious boys was at the top of the list. She also provided their family (and sometimes relatives, visitors, and neighbors) with the best divinely prepared meals. She made their home and anything else she touched fit for royalty. She somehow transformed their backyard into an enchanted garden with her sheer creative ingenuity and a few household items. If her contributions weren't already enough, she even refused a servant when Bereket offered to find her one to assist around the house, insisting that: "*A woman is the maker of her own home.*" Denkenesh was the epitome of womanhood.

As Denkenesh drifted off into deep thought about her early experiences with the health and wellness practices of her ancestors, she saw Bereket carry a large bundle of special wood into the newly constructed *Gojo*. The wood, called "*Wayra*" in Amharic, produced the "*Weybatis*" meaning, 'smoky essence' which was selected due to its many therapeutic properties. In addition to *weybatis*, the bark and leaves of the *wayra* tree were boiled in hot water to make a medicinal tea to assist with upset stomachs. It is also blended with other barks and herbs to soothe cramps, disinfect cuts or wounds, relieve joint pain, and clean or detoxify the lungs, among many other therapeutic benefits.

Denkenesh specifically requested that Bereket place her *Gojo* in the backyard so that it would be nestled alongside the veranda for the perfect balance of privacy and convenience. She also wanted it to be in close proximity to the grand, old Juniper tree, the favorite feature of her garden. The grand Juniper tree was located in the center of the yard; those beautiful Juniper leaves stretched over everything offered wonderful shade on hot summer days. There was something peaceful, calming, and reassuring about Juniper trees. They made her feel connected to the Creator as the designer of beautiful things like trees.

All of this – the *Gojo*, the Juniper Tree, and the *weybatis* – reminded Denkenesh of her Grandmother Selamawet, whose own *Gojo* is situated in the backyard of her house also near a large Juniper tree. But, almost everything she loved about life seemed to be connected to her grandmother, for that matter.

Bereket was keenly aware of how much Denkenesh missed her village, but more important to her was taking *weybatis* in total relaxation and comfort where she lived now with her husband. *Weybatis* was a time set aside for women to get respite from everyday life. Women often smoked themselves together and offered support to one another as friends. But things were different now that Denkenesh and Bereket had joined as one through marriage. They both sacrificed the old and familiar to establish a blossoming new life together – a life of hope, laughter, and promise. The high cost did not matter to either of them, even though that meant leaving her family behind to establish a new home and life in Bereket's village.

And for this devotion, Bereket felt that the least he could do was make it possible for his wife to have this luxury. So, he built Denkenesh her own *Gojo*, acquired a years' supply of *Wayra* for the *Weybatis*, and gathered the vessels required to store her inventory of ingredients for what he thought of as a sort of *monthly wellness ceremony* just for women.

Bereket was honored to be married to Denkenesh. He felt proud that his wife hailed from the legendary women of Wolo. The women of her bloodline were hailed among the most beautiful, compassionate, and highly sought-after women in all of Ethiopia. Even more, respect was bestowed on them for being the premiere experts of *Weybatis*, one of the oldest and most powerful therapeutic wellness practices touted for improving health and enhancing feminine sensuality. Being the originators of the *Weybatis,* which is sometimes referred to as "*Kokabatis*" has truly made them renowned throughout Ethiopia. Their skill with this traditional form of healing has perpetuated feminine essence, natural beauty, and womb health as an art and science influencing women around the world.

Since the times of Queen Makeda of Sheba, the women of Wolo have engaged in *Weybatis*, smoking themselves to induce feminine wellness as routine self-care. Their ingenuity with *Weybatis* led to a sacred healing tradition steeped in medicinal benefits used throughout Ethiopia by women of all ages to treat many womb related conditions, including, but not limited to irregular periods, back pain, menstrual pain, joint stiffness, hormonal imbalance, vaginal tears, infections, abdominal cramping, and abnormal vaginal discharges.

It was even used to increase female libido and treat infertility in women. In fact, Denkenesh wanted to smoke for a very special reason. She and Bereket wanted to have another child. It was time to prepare her body to conceive and carry a third child, which they both hoped would be their very first daughter.

Since the days of old, the women of her family took great pains to keep the tradition of vaginal smoking alive. Being direct descendants of the Queen of Sheba, who also engaged in *Weybatis*, they took the honor of passing this sacred wisdom of healing along to their daughters. Each successive generation of girls would develop into powerful, healthy, fertile women who continued the art of healing for beauty, health, and wellness as a sacred member of this family line.

My sacred daughters, you see, every matriarch – whether she is the grandmother or a mother- around the world wants her daughter to be healthy and beautiful. It makes me so happy to fill these pages with beautiful knowledge for you to read. This way, I, too, am taking the honor of passing along the sacred wisdom of healing traditions to my promising granddaughters and to a long line of descendants that I hope will do the same.

Okay, let's continue...

Now that she had her own *Gojo* again, Denkenesh could pass the tradition onto any future daughters she would have of her own. It would begin once the female child came of age, as indicated by the start of her "*Yawre Abeba*," meaning 'monthly flower,' which was a beautiful metaphor to denote her menstrual cycle.

Denkenesh never forgot that special day when her own *Yawre Abeba* or monthly cycle began because the response her mother gave was full of tenderness and kindness. When the bright red spots stained her new *kemese*, a white dress made of pure cotton, Denkenesh was filled with worry. She thought she might get in trouble for ruining it. When she finally mustered the courage to inform her mother about the situation she found herself in, she directed her mother's attention toward the stain on the back of her dress by shyly pointing her finger at the spot without saying a word. Although she wanted to explain that she was innocent of any wrongdoing, the words she needed would not leave her mouth. That is, because she didn't know *what* to say. All of this was unexpected. But to Denkenesh's great surprise, her mother simply gave her a loving smile. With tears that swelled up in her piercing dark eyes, she patiently explained to Denkenesh, "*It is coming from your 'Dabo'. It means you're growing up now.*"

All her life, Denkenesh had only known one word to describe her vagina, and that word was "*Dabo.*" Although there was an official term for it, no one ever uttered the Amharic word, "*emese*" – it was too impolite to speak about a woman's sacred part in such terms. It is just too direct. Culturally speaking, the custom was to say "*Dabo*" instead, and that is the way it remained generation after generation.

"*Dabo*," meaning "*beautiful bread*," is a wonderful metaphor that serves as a perfect description to communicate this sacred aspect of womanhood. Not only was it polite, but it also signified something sacred – something that is necessary and full of life. *Dabo* is a loving expression that speaks to the aspect of womanhood that should make every woman feel safe, cherished, and desired. Like a beautiful loaf of bread, our wombs should be fresh, warm, organic, wholesome, and maintain the perfect level of moisture.

My beloved granddaughters, you will soon discover that the practice of *weybatis* is what helps facilitate that reality for women even today, just as it has during ancient times. Keep what I have said about *Dabo* in the back of your mind as we continue with the story of Denkenesh.

Shortly after her *yawre abeba,* or monthly flower, completed its first cycle, which was about three days later, Denkenesh was escorted by her grandmother, Selamawet, to the *Gojo* located behind her home. There she observed in silence as her grandmother made the preparation for her first *Weybatis* experience.

Her grandmother told her that she wanted to wait until the sun began to set before lighting the wood and placing it inside of the "*gudegade*," which is a pear-shaped hole dug about one foot deep into the fresh earth with the wide part at the bottom. In the meantime, Grandmother helped Denkenesh lather herself in the "*kebi*," or a thick butter made from fresh cow milk. Her grandmother had already infused the *kebi* with powdered lavender called "*addes*" in the Amharic language.

At the setting sun, Denkenesh was draped from the neck down in a new "*gabi*," which is a large, heavy blanket made with 100% cotton. At sunset, Grandmother ignited the special wood, which formed into a billowing, aromatic "*weybatis*" or smoky essence from the *wayra* wood. Her grandmother then directed Denkenesh to sit on top of the low stool called a "*duka*" that was situated directly over the smoke-filled hole so that Denkenesh's womb was right above the smoke. The "*duka*" or stool was custom made just for *weybatis* and crafted from the *wayra* or the same special wood that formed the *weybatis* or smoky essence. It had a large hole cut into the seat so the smoke could rise through from the hole beneath or "*gudegade*" and be directed to her exposed womb entrance. With the help of the blanket, however, all the smoky essence was captured, and eventually, her entire body was smoked, including her feet which were nestled comfortably over two smaller *duka* or stools. These stools were also handcrafted from *wayra* and shaped to a curve that supports the back of the feet, which allows the womb to relax and open. The purpose of this was to increase blood flow and support her back.

The practice of *weybatis* promotes the release of toxins from the skin by facilitating the profuse sweating of the entire body. Grandmother Selamawet reserved a large portion of the *kebi* or butter for the crown melting. This is done by placing a large scoop of the butter over the head and allowing it to slowly melt down into the hair, scalp, face, ears, and neck. As a result, the eyes, mouth, and nose were moisturized in the milky substance. This was Denkenesh's first *weybatis*. It lasted for an hour and left her feeling wholesome, rejuvenated, and pure. Remembering how the warm aromatic smoking of her womb always made her feel so beautiful, soft, energized, and completely renewed, put a beaming smile on her face.

Just when she was finishing that beautiful thought, Denkenesh was summoned by Bereket to see the beautiful structure he had just completed. Beaming with joy, Denkenesh went outside to finally see the finished *Gojo*. She could already smell the weybatis in the **air**. To her, it was the **earthy** scent of *Divine SelfQare*.

Chapter 8

Total Body Alignment

My sacred granddaughters and grandsons, before I begin with everything that I have in store for you here, I just want to thank you for being with me on this beautiful and enlightening journey. The work that I have put into *The Divine SelfQare Strategy* would have meant nothing if it didn't have all your precious souls as my readers.

Up to this point, I have spent a great deal of time and attention on various topics related to Divine Health and Freedom. We began with laying the foundation of family legacy with its roots deeply embedded in healing and health practices as reflected through the lives of our matriarchs.

Starting with my Grandmother Betty, Great-grandmother Lena Mae, and Great-great-grandmother Rebecca, we reviewed several stories illustrating their determination to survive, regardless of the conditions. Time and time again, these matriarchs taught us how to become a force to be reckoned with. With the knowledge they passed down to us – their resilience comes as no surprise.

Next, we focused on the collective brilliance of key historical figures, including the honorable Frederick Douglas, QM Harriet Tubman, QM Harriet Jacobs, and Dr. Martin L. King Jr. to provide us with irrefutable contextual evidence about everything that the *Divine SelfQare Strategy* stands for. Other historically significant healers such as elders Gus Smith and Sally Brown also played a significant role in shedding light on the genius that our ancestors were equipped with - especially with respect to healing and natural medicine.

The reason I can imagine myself sitting surrounded by you, my beautiful grandchildren, teaching you the ways of our elders is that the foundation of our health principles is rooted in their life experiences and success strategies. Undoubtedly, this shows us the connection between freedom and health while revealing that both of these are rooted in our Divine Connection to the Most High. The Most High is the superior source responsible for giving us not only the five elements, but the knowledge of how to use them through the science of *trans-physics*.

My beloved children, let me say it once again, the very solid foundation that makes it possible to see the force that fuels our efforts to achieve freedom and secure remarkable health is *Divine Intention*. All life goals are pursued by way of intention. Whether we harm or help others in the process of achieving them is dependent upon our desire. Either we are in alignment with the will of the Most High or opposed to the rules of *Divine Justice* and Spiritual Balance.

When there is alignment, the earth prospers in harmony with humanity. It promotes growth, healing, and renewal throughout the world. That being said, out of the several teachings that this book holds, I want you to remember the truth behind the Divine Intention. Look inside your heart every time you set out on a path to fulfill your life's goals. This way, you will always be in harmony with the environment that the Most High has so graciously created for you.

But beloved, if we as a people are out of alignment with the Most High's will in the pursuit of our life's goals, it can result in disruptions to growth and innovation, the destruction of nature, a decline of the global population and health, and, worse, the deprivation of freedom. Hence, to protect our freedom, innovation, and the earth's brimming life, divine alignment is key.

But the question that remains here is, *why*? Why did I choose to invest my time in this book? What was the purpose of it all?

Well, in my efforts to grasp this concept my beloved children, I had to return to our sacred and ancient wisdom of healing, and as a faithful daughter of the Most High, I asked the All-Knowing One for answers. I wanted to know how it was possible for our people to survive through four hundred years of political and medical tyranny. A part of me wanted to understand what kind of power was bestowed on our ancestors that made them so resilient despite everything we have gone through collectively.

My mind has always been perplexed about two critical extremes. It was astonishing to learn about the cruel operations on the innocent bodies of men and women in the form of medical exploitation, on the one hand, and complete medical neglect on the other. What was the Divine Strength that our people were accessing in order to survive? Whatever it was, I wanted to capture it, study it, make sense of it, and preserve it in writing for you beloved and for the generations to come. And, if possible, to make it last for all time.

Understanding everything our ancestors' endured throughout history led me on a journey of my own. I was guided by Divine Imagination to envision another time, life, and reality - one beyond the period that began our journey in this country. One that led me beyond the shock of the brutal experiments that tore into the dignity and ripped the very flesh of the sons and daughters of the Most High.

But more importantly, I wanted a way to overcome the dent in our history left when the medical profession supported people like Dr. J. Marion Sims, who operated on the tortured bodies of Anaracha, Lucy and Betsy, three enslaved women. He did so without their permission, without compensation to them, and worse, without mercy for them.

For too many years the unimaginable pain and mutilation that these women had to endure have haunted my mind. Yet, it's not just history. One can't ignore that there are potentially millions of reported and unreported cases of medical malpractice perpetuated in hospitals, clinics, private labs, and undisclosed test facilities to this day that still deprive men and women of their health and lives. Could it be the *vestiges* of a disturbing medical past originating with slavery that resurfaces periodically?

In response to my request for answers, the Most High ushered me into a series of events that ranged from chance encounters and spontaneous conversations, to divine insights and revelations. Sometimes this knowledge took the form of old songs and stories narrated to me. Others came in the form of historical records, which unveiled knowledge about us women, the needs of our bodies, and valuable ancient healing techniques meant to address those needs as practiced to this day by select women throughout the African Diaspora. Alongside this body of knowledge that I share with you today my grandchildren, unfolded many mysteries that helped to simply reveal what I believe amounts to the sacred healing science of *Total Body Alignment*.

Before we get into understanding the art of *Total Body Alignment*, here is a little something to help you navigate through everything I am going to talk about in the chapter.

The Divine SelfQare Strategy

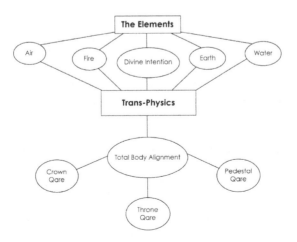

The Art Of Total Body Alignment | Grounded | Centered | Elevated

My beloved children, at this point, you must be wondering what *Total Body Alignment* has to do with Divine Health, the Science of *Trans-physics*, and the Elements or *Divine SelfQare*? Well, everything we discussed before informs the lessons I will impart to you now.

Trust me, my precious granddaughters, and grandsons, it will all make sense when we begin.

Let's start with this, have you ever considered the possibility that trees in nature correlate to a woman's body? Think about it - all the similarities. Now, use your Divine Imagination to take a brief journey with me.

> *Close your eyes and imagine a strong, tall, beautiful cedar tree as if it were standing erect directly in front of you right now. Imagine that you place your body right next to the tree so that your feet are standing right above the exposed roots.*
>
> *On such a large outlying tree, the exposed roots almost mirror the spreading branches above, providing balance and symmetry just like your outstretched hands and standing feet. Throughout the ages, interpretations of the tree as a symbol have sprouted, however, the fundamental elements remain - a flourishing tree with outstretched branches and strong roots embedded into the earth.*
>
> *I want you to feel how sturdy the roots are, even as the tops of them can be seen surfacing above the ground like the top part of your feet are visible while the bottoms are in contact with the earth.*

Notice the long bark of the tree? Rub your hands along its length as far as you can reach, and then wrap your arms around it to cover as much circumference as possible. Now, as you examine the vertical shape as it rises above the roots, observe how the bark seems to center itself in the air and how it connects the roots in the soil located at the very bottom to the branches and its leaves way above, without ever letting them touch each other.

Now, compare this function to your own core. Do you notice how your torso is similar to the bark and how it connects your grounded feet to your arms, neck, and head, yet they never touch each other either? Like the bark of the cedar tree, your waist, chest, and hips play a similar role and maintain a similar cylindrical shape.

Next, tilt your head up to the sky to observe the long branches and leaves at the top of the cedar wood tree as they reach for the heavens; now stretch your two arms up and out just like the cedar wood tree branches.

When your feet are planted firmly onto the earth you feel a sense of groundedness much like the cedar tree is deeply rooted in the soil. When your womb is in harmony and stabilized at the core above your wide hips, strong legs and below your firm, straight waist, and chest you feel centered like the core or bark of the cedar wood tree. When your neck, head, and hair are up in the air looking for inspiration in the clouds you feel elevated like the branches and leaves of the cedar tree outstretched toward the sun.

> *So, essentially this grounding, centering, and elevating aspect of your being is what you have in common with the cedar tree and just about every other healthy tree on earth for that matter. Both you, as a woman and the cedar in your mind's eyes are experiencing Divine Alignment. What total nature alignment is to the tree is Total Body Alignment for you. Now open your eyes...*

I want you to know that I chose the cedar wood tree because it's special for many reasons. It is a sacred tree full of bounty and purpose. The special connection between people and trees can be seen in cultures all over the world, even going back to ancient times. As we admire the cedar wood tree today and understand the importance of its role in relaying the symmetry of *Total Body Alignment*, so did many people before us. The Ancient Africans used the oil extracted from the bark for embalming practices. The Ancient Mesopotamians used resin from the cedar wood tree as a base for paint, and for other cultures it held spiritual and religious significance as well.

The thing that resonates with us about the cedar tree as Daughters of the Most High is that it is commonly associated with fertility and abundance. Amongst many different cultures and nations fertility is an important concept. For us as Daughters of the Most High, not only does it speak to our sacred duty to conceive, carry, and bring forth life to perpetuate humanity, but it also symbolizes our inherent gift of Divine Creativity.

We express fertility in many ways beyond physical labor and birthing children. We also give birth to ideas, business concepts, inventions, art, and resolutions to life's many problems. We literally birth humanity but theoretically, we also give birth to the *humanities*.

Perhaps, something that I wish for this book is that it would serve as a wholesome journey that allows you to educate yourself with its anecdotes, but at the same time, equip your mind with its holistic analysis. As a grandmother, I can read a million stories to you, my beloved granddaughters and grandsons, but they will only be worth it if you, my grandchildren, are able to extract something useful from them.

I want you to be able to interrelate the concepts highlighted in this book to create a deeper understanding of how the tools that are used to facilitate the *Divine SelfQare Strategy* exist around us. These very tools - **Air, Fire, Earth**, and **Water**, plus **Divine Intent** - had empowered women and men across the globe to thrive even before we were born.

Denkenesh | Woman Of Divine Imagination

Do you remember the beautiful story of Denkenesh? I want you to recall that at the center of her garden stood a sacred juniper tree. This is by design. It is to remind us that we are connected to nature. That what you see as a healthy tree is bountiful, giving fruit, full of life, lush green leaves that provide shade, and a strong healthy bark rooted deeply below the ground in proportions similar to what your eyes can see above. Doesn't that astonish?

The top of the tree is always reaching for the creator of heaven and earth, always evidencing the invisible gift of its sacred relationship with the Most High. Through its bountiful, abundant yield of seasonal flowers, seeds, blossoms, and fruit it encapsulates the essence of everything that the Most High has lovingly designed for us. The Creator supplies what is needed below the earth where the tree is nurtured, watered, and replenished.

Likewise, we as women show ourselves beautiful to the world, but this beauty is the product of the unseen work we too must do to elevate our minds, balance our spirit, and nourish, hydrate, and replenish our bodies. We do this with the tools given to us by the Most High in the form of **air, fire, earth,** and **water** – through the science *of trans-physics* to experience *Total Body Alignment.*

So, what role does the lovely Denkenesh play, my children? Well, Denkenesh is a woman of fiction – *a product of Divine Imagination.* Yet, her story is the perfect depiction of several realistic relationships and wellness routines practiced by the women of Ethiopia long, long ago. In fact, my sacred daughters, I created this story after consulting with knowledgeable Ethiopian women like Yeshimebet, so that after this labor or love, I could share with you some of the important, ancient aspects of *Divine SelfQare.*

This is the importance of stories. They paint a picture of history, because multigenerational stories and anecdotes passed down from our ancestors are meant to help shape how each new generation perceives things. Let me ask you a simple question, my precious children. If some unfortunate soul lost a decade worth of memories, what do you think that person would do to relearn everything that was missed? I think you know the answer. Read literature! They'd read books, newspapers, or any other form of journalism that captures the essence of what shapes a decade.

That being said, what is written history? Is it not our perspectives all combined into opinions, critiques, and analysis? In this manner, the story of Denkenesh is a beautiful piece of literature from a time when *Divine SelfQare* was held so close to every woman's heart that it patterned the rhythm of her feet. It is meant to send you back to a time when chemicals, unnatural ingredients, ridiculous body images, and processes to maintain them did not exist. Women were free from thoughts of these things. They lived in complete harmony with nature because they chose to protect, cleanse, nourish, and heal themselves using the power of the five elements the Most High gifted to them.

So, Denkenesh, a woman of fiction, serves as a beacon of hope and possibility for you and all that I wish for you, my beautiful granddaughters. Our matriarchs drew power from their beliefs to form and influence our perspectives. Similarly, you will one day draw wisdom and strength from your experiences (like the one you are having while reading this book) to shape future generations. Perhaps this is the reason why history, symbols, anecdotes, and stories are so important. They serve as metaphors for life.

My beautiful grandchildren, I want nothing but the very best for you and your sense of health, wellness, love and security for generations to come. Although the world we find ourselves in today is far different from that of Denkenesh's in so many ways. Regardless, the loving supportive relationships we saw illustrated throughout the story between a woman and her family, her Creator, her home environment, her community, and her relationship with self, is something worth reviewing and in my opinion working toward. Let Denkenesh and her beautiful story serve as a marker for the quality of life one can achieve if they adhere to the *Divine SelfQare Strategy* and strive for *Total Body Alignment* in their lives.

Denkenesh | Cycle of Divine Womanhood

Now, let's focus on Denkenesh and how her relationships nurture and validate all aspects of femininity. Undoubtedly, women are more intuitive when it comes to establishing and maintaining relationships. However, with Denkenesh, we see a direct relationship between her spiritual and physical wellness, and how that translates into a woman living her best life. This becomes highly possible and can be evidenced by what we can observe about her childhood.

Denkenesh was groomed by highly spiritual women to care for her body as a temple. A temple is a sacred place where one communes with the creator. Notice how gently and lovingly Denkenesh's mother spoke to her about her *"yawre abeba"* or *"monthly flower"*? This is because one of the first lessons a young woman should learn is how to relate to her feminine process. It also reinforces my reasons for writing this book for you, sweet granddaughters of mine, so that one day this labor of love can serve as a compilation of essential lessons that every girl needs to learn from her matriarchs.

Speaking of important lessons, the menstrual cycle is perhaps one of the most important ones! It is something to be welcomed and celebrated. Without it, life cannot continue, and humanity will not perpetuate itself. Even though it is understandable why some people would find it loathsome, it is important to understand the significance of this beautiful sign of fertility. A menstrual cycle isn't supposed to be painful or disgusting. Instead, it is to be anticipated, monitored, and accommodated. My sacred granddaughters, you might wonder what I mean by accommodated. Well, I mean that, as women, we should know our cycles. We should understand it, measure it, analyze it, and most importantly, anticipate it because it is a sacred gift from the Most High that most women take for granted.

Denkenesh's mother was relieved when Denkenesh started her cycle. Like for most mothers and grandmothers around the world, a daughter who receives her first period is a pretty big deal, something to be appreciated and celebrated. She spoke to Denkenesh in a loving and reassuring tone and ushered her into the blossoming world of womanhood. That is what the cycle of Divine Womanhood represents. Her grandmother also played an important role in this cycle as she taught Denkenesh that women have a strategy for managing the health of their bodies.

She also emphasized how the start of Denkenesh's cycle meant that it was time for her to be inducted into the concept of feminine health and wellness as employed by her people. This meant that as a woman who hailed from the legendary women of Wolo, she was to relish in the science and wisdom of vaginal wellness using the elements of **air, fire, earth,** and **water** to induce cleansing, relaxation, and rejuvenation after the full completion of her menstrual cycle. Her cycle marked the beginning of a new life, aligned with a Divine Purpose, to birth humanity and become a symbol of divine creativity and strength that enables the human race to live on. With the gift of fertility, a woman is given the power to grow life inside her womb - something the opposite sex can never experience naturally. She becomes a Divine Vessel full of the strength, knowledge, power, love, and faith while carrying the hope of her people onward to the future.

Unfortunately, many girls around the world are taught how to reject a key aspect of their bodies as well as the biological mechanism that gives rise to life. It could be labeled as a failure of the education system or lack of awareness in female matriarchs. But, somehow, some of us tend not to honor ourselves and the hormonal fluctuations that occur naturally in our bodies, and so we remain detached from our bodies or how to tune into our own inner rhythms.

Women are rarely ever shown the sacredness, creativity, and wisdom that is embedded in their rhythmic monthly cycle — the feminine cycle — or how to embrace this period of cleansing and renewal, which is why the *Divine SelfQare Strategy* is my gift to you.

If we live in alignment with the seasons of our cycle, stop rejecting it, and actually understand which of our strengths and qualities are highlighted during each phase, we can become more productive, more at ease in our own bodies, and more confident, productive, and powerful women as a whole.

Beautiful granddaughters of mine, this feminine essence that I speak of is what epitomizes a woman, especially when she is perceived by those who love and care for her. This Divine Knowledge lays the early foundation for how she treats herself and how she should also expect to be treated by others who respect her strengths and vulnerabilities as a woman. It is no wonder that her husband, Bereket, had such a deep appreciation for Denkenesh; he knew how cherished and important she was to her birth family. He held nothing but a desire to maintain the most optimal levels of care and respect for his wife's physical needs as her husband. In doing so, he also fed and nurtured her spirit just as he knew that Denkenesh had experienced with her birth family. It was his job, as her husband, to facilitate the resources needed to continue her healing and wellness traditions and he did this with an open heart.

In return, Denkenesh was able to meet the demands of being a wife, mother, and productive member of a large community. She was the manager of her own valuable resources. Her desire was to establish a kingdom with her husband and raise healthy children in a loving, beautiful environment that reminded her of her birth family's values, home, and upbringing. She was adored by Bereket and her sons. She now wished to ensure that she could pass along her wisdom of motherhood along to a daughter, just like how I wish to do for you, beloved granddaughters.

The point of relating this to you my grandchildren, is to show you how integral relationships are to our sense of wellness and how they should always be factored into *Divine SelfQare*. Without healthy, productive, and loving relationships with those we trust and to whose care we are entrusted, *Divine SelfQare* is difficult to achieve.

My beautiful granddaughters, I want so many wonderful things for you: a life of abundance, health, family, safety, and protection. I want respect for you. I want you to respect yourself. I want you to recognize that in your youth, you are like a delicate flower. You need time to blossom. Don't rush the process but allow yourself to take root in strength until you transform like a sacred cedar tree that has outstretched branches, is fertile, fruitful and connected at the roots to a solid past. These roots connect you to an ancestry that was not only powerful, but also a part of the Divine Kingdom that the Most High saw fit to plant and bless with life – life that is both temporal physically and eternal spiritually.

Denkenesh | Exemplar of Divine Relationships

Beautiful granddaughters of mine, my hope is that when you read this you will get a sense of how simple, satisfying, and beautiful life can be when our relationships align with our *Divine SelfQare* Practices to produce Divine Health. Through Denkenesh's story, I hope to shed light on the origins of *Divine SelfQare* and illustrate the five pillars in the form of relationships that foster Divine Health.

As a *Divine SelfQare* Practitioner, who helps women from all walks of life, I often see how women sometimes have less than optimal results in the area of womb and body wellness because of the toxic environment and people that they have to engage with daily. Sometimes these experiences are nothing short of demoralizing. A woman may want to live a better, healthier, natural life. She may want to improve, but she may have a spouse or children who devalue her and therefore devalue any ideas that are proffered by her to benefit her physical, mental, and spiritual health.

I recently encountered a situation where a woman acquired my *ThroneQare Steam Station* and was all excited about starting her journey. But her husband believed this sacred and special work towards an improved lifestyle to be silly. He wrote it, and me off, as the maker of this Total Body Alignment system, as some kind of a "*quack.*" To state it frankly, he was not going to be an ally along her journey to wellness. And this, too, is tragic.

But my prayer, hope, and strong desire are that this type of scenario will not ever be your experience or reality. Once you grasp the ideas in this book, you will realize that the *Divine SelfQare Strategy* is just as much about the quality of our relationships as women as it is about the womb and *Total Body Alignment*. Denkenesh's life is one filled with loving, supportive, affirming bonds that create productive relationships and maintain health. Denkenesh feels safe, valued, and protected by those she loves – namely her mother, grandmother, husband, children, community, and of course, her *Creator*, the Most High. In addition to that, Denkenesh lives in an environment that is conducive to her expression of creativity, her gifts as a mother, wife, creative expressionist, and conveyer of her culture through cleanliness.

I hope to shed light on the ways her life could serve as an ideal situation – not to dictate that you live exactly as Denkenesh lived but to analyze your relationship with yourself, your family, your environment, and more importantly, with your Creator.

Her story and the knowledge you extract from it isn't a bad place to start the conversation by any stretch of the imagination. You should feel free to read the story to your spouse, children, parents, extended family and loved ones to raise the question as to whether we are really doing the best we can to build up, lift up, and support one another for optimal health and life's true purpose as healers, supporters, providers and protectors.

The relationships highlighted in the Denkenesh story pave the path for us to explore the definition of healthy relationships. They become guidance for us to learn how to strengthen the sanctity of our relationships, not just with the people around us, but with the Most High. Being in alignment with the divine principles of the Creator can bring immense joy because then can you be in harmony with nature, apply principles of divine law, and be thankful for the life that has been given to you. The fact that our matriarchs had the strength to fight off the forces of sickness, untimely death, violence, and bondage time and time again is proof that giving honor to the Most High for the gift of endurance has a gracious return.

My grandchildren, how else do you think that our ancestors wielded the elements as their weapons against the oppressive forces that continuously sought to bind them? One cannot deny that these wise men and women had strength, faith, and confidence in themselves and a solid relationship with the Most High.

Similarly, the story of Denkenesh also points in the same direction. Let's further explore these relationship dynamics, my beloved granddaughters and grandsons. Each and every principle that you conceptualize through reading her story is real. So, my task in this segment of the book is to convey two big things to you. The first is how Divine Health is dependent upon our quality of, access to, and management of five core types of relationships – namely the ones we have with ourselves, family, environment, community, and the Most High. The second is that the origin of *Divine SelfQare* is rooted in something ancient, divine, and organic, connected to the oldest people in the world – particularly women of African descent, who have been exercising their gift of healing since the beginning of time.

Denkenesh's experience is a sweet way of conveying the marriage of these two concepts in a succinct but hopefully engaging and interesting way. That being said, my precious granddaughters read this chapter with an inquisitive mind and ask yourself questions about your own world of experiences. Ponder upon the different areas of her life and ways of living and compare them to your own life and lived experiences. How are they different, better, or similar? Can you find ways to improve your communications with others in ways that help you confidently express your needs and desires like Denkenesh?

All of these things and more are what I hope to spark in your hearts, sweet daughters of mine. Because in doing so, you can set your life apart from the pain and confusion that so many others have endured over the ages simply because of the rigors of time, the tragedy of wars, and ignorance about our cultures and traditions. More than 400 years of physical and mental bondage in this country alone, but also in other places around the world, have taken a toll on our people. The amount of loss we have collectively suffered becomes the core reason for us to seek out that which is righteous and worthy of reclaiming in the name of health, wellness, and heritage. Read on now! There is so much that your grandmother wants to reveal to you...

Denkenesh | Pillars of Divine Health

My granddaughters, as I have stated before, this story, and this entire book is just as much about Divine Health as it is about *Divine SelfQare*. Here, we are going to delve into what I call *"The Five Pillars Of Divine Health."* These pillars help you understand the basis of healthy relationships. I have discovered that relationships have a direct impact on the ability to feel mental, spiritual and physical wellness and to possess the energy needed to pursue the path of Divine Purpose.

As you can imagine, Divine Health and *SelfQare* are much more involved than eating healthy and engaging in exercise. It is about finding the right balance between your needs and what the environment you find yourself around has to offer.

Nutrition and exercise can fulfill a certain aspect of health, but it seldom has an impact on your spiritual and psychological health the way *Total Body Alignment* and these other crucial pillars do when used in conjunction with nutrition and exercise.

In Denkenesh's story, we get to see several sacred relationships: Denkenesh as a mother, a child and grandchild, a citizen, a daughter of the Most High, and last but not least, a wife.

Pillar One: Personal Health & Wellness

Denkenesh is setting aside time to protect and preserve her sense of mental, physical, and spiritual well-being and personal autonomy in a space intentionally designed for that purpose.

Pillar Two: Total Body Alignment

Denkenesh is engaging in a health practice that supports and honors the importance of the three key aspects of womanhood that align the total body, which begins with the head, the womb, and the feet. Other body parts then also become part of her *Divine SelfQare* and wellness routine.

Pillar Three: Strategic Personal Planning

Denkenesh is designing a meaningful life intentionally. She co-creates the desires of her heart with her husband, Bereket. Together they decide to pursue their desires to expand their family, hoping to have a daughter this time around. Note how Denkenesh takes measures in advance to prepare her body for childbirth.

Pillar Four: Cultural Continuity

Denkenesh is reflecting on the beautiful lessons learned from her grandmother and mother about *Divine SelfQare* and Wellness. She aspires to have her own daughter, who will be taught these principles as well.

Pillar Five: Divine Resources

Denkenesh is pursuing wellness and has all the physical resources she needs to continue her *Divine SelfQare Strategies*. She also has another vital resource. She has *love*. In fact, Denkenesh is fortunate to not only spring from a loving family that engages in healthy forms of communication, but she is blessed to be in a relationship with a man who adores, protects, and honors her needs and desires. Bereket strives to supply everything necessary to support Denkenesh's physical, spiritual, and emotional needs.

Now beloved, let's delve deeper into the meaning behind each important aspect of the Denkenesh story. This will help you better conceptualize the assets that every woman needs and should have in her life at some point or another to feel and be as healthy and whole as possible.

My sacred daughters, as we continue our discussion, I want you to use your Divine Imagination again. Envision Denkenesh in the village of her youth so that you can see the evolution of her journey as it relates to Divine Health.

We'll start with revisiting what it means to have and pursue Divine Health...

Recall, precious ones, that Divine Health is a state that we should constantly work to achieve. It means to:

- *be in excellent physical condition*
- *to possess a sound mind*
- *to experience spiritual balance at any age*

Like most ideals, affirmations, and beliefs, this seems pretty simple in theory, but in today's world, it may not be that easy to accomplish in reality. I imagine that by the time you are old enough to conceptualize the lessons in this book, the world will have become more complex than it is now, making the pursuit of Divine Health even more challenging. For each passing day, the rising dependency on chemicals, drugs, unnecessary technology, and over-the-top beauty standards, the world has made society a problematic place for us as Daughters of the Most High to thrive in.

But, that really is the purpose of the book. *The Divine SelfQare Strategy* is meant to provide you with a holistic guide to the mind and body, powered by the grace of the Most High. So, at the end of the day, you can have the strength and tools you will need to live above and beyond the superficial things of life.

It is upon my shoulders to have the foresight to recognize your need and offer you a compass or a roadmap to guide your energies and help align you with the beautiful things life has to offer. I seek to help you possess the right knowledge, wisdom, and understanding about the secrets I am sharing on *Divine SelfQare* and how to pursue Divine Health using **A.F.E.W.** tools just as efficiently as our ancestors have done throughout history under circumstances far more challenging.

The question that we derive here, my children, is why do you need Divine Health in the first place? Isn't it just enough to have good health?

To answer this, I would like to shed light on how Divine Health leads to Divine Purpose, and Divine Purpose is what connects us to our spiritual source - the Most High, who is the Creator of all life.

Being a woman of Divine Purpose means being connected to our source - the Most High, who is beyond the finite realm of time. It means being able to call on our Creator, who is greater than all, who is beyond time, who protects and provides a place for us in the great scheme of life, and who enables us to experience what is called *now*. We have emerged, unaware, by the grace of the Most High from a period called *history* and we will emerge, by the grace of the Most High, into an experience called the *future*.

Knowing this, as I have discovered, gives you the motivation to do something for someone you may never meet (like future generations of people who will prayerfully descend from me through my son, Zakur - and yes, even you one day). That is what motivated and inspired me to write this book for those I may never have the privilege of meeting in person. Our Grand Matriarchs, Rebecca, Lena Mae, and Betty planted this desire within me with their memorable stories about life. Perhaps, one day, I'll get to do the same for you, beloved. Always remember, no matter where or when we exist in the world, we are connected, my sacred grandchildren.

For instance, I am compelled to tell you about the great feats of heroism, the great acts of defiance, and the great mastery of Divine Health and *Divine SelfQare* that our collective ancestors achieved. You know them well now, divine practitioners like QM Harriet Tubman and QM Harriet Jacobs, and the divine knowers and activists, like Elder Frederick Douglas and Dr. Martin Luther King, whom I told you about in the earlier chapters of the book, along with our personal families who are counted among these great people. A common thread among them all were their able bodies that allowed them to overcome the obstacles to experience physical perseverance, spiritual balance, and a sound mind.

There are direct barriers to having the kind of mental peace required for a sound mind. Wouldn't you agree that slavery, Jim Crow laws, and other forms of mental oppression were among them? Imagine being unable to have the freedom to think independently, or plan a life of abundance and prosperity, or choose the places you will go, live, and explore with your family! This obstructs mental wellbeing.

Imagine the whips, beatings, and the cruelty of slavery. It's hard to visit the oppressive conditions of the Jim Crow South, even in the mind, because this is where the brutality of racism was meted out more violently than in the Jane Crow North, where it often happened benignly.

Grandchildren, do you believe that any of us *today* could have a spiritual life, full of balance and mental bliss under those unimaginably horrific conditions? Of course, my granddaughters and sons, you already know that the answer to this question is *no*. Just thinking or reading about such traumatizing conditions weighs heavily upon the mind and spirit. All of this is said to remind you that *Divine SelfQare* is a precious gift and a blessing to have today. It is a practice vastly different from anything you've previously understood. It is not a spa day with the girls at the local nail shop where you line up to receive the typical pedicure, manicure, or eyebrow shaping. It is not about removing hair or adding paint to toes and fingernails, nor is it about subjecting yourself to hours of invasive procedures by undergoing heat, cold, pressings or external suctioning to contour the body.

My beautiful daughters, I pray that you never spend an hour of your life wondering how to please others, how to get others to love you, how to get others to approve of you, or pursue beauty standards that are out of alignment with nature. Instead, my hope is that your life choices begin with searching yourself first and then acting on what you need and what you want through self-actualization. Self-actualization is just another way of describing the pursuit of Divine Purpose. This is the opposite of selfishness. It is about you taking full responsibility for something only you can be responsible for – that is, your own healthcare, healing and wellbeing. No one can bring you closer to this goal than you and the Most High.

Divine SelfQare is rooted in three principles...

The first is that Divine Health is your birthright and that it is vital to the fulfillment of your Divine Purpose.

The second is that your body is a sacred temple that requires you to have a strong foundation that is connected to your feet; an unobstructed threshold that is connected to your womb; and, a level dome which is symbolic of your head. Another way of thinking of these three aspects of a woman's body metaphorically is as a *crown*, a *throne*, and a *pedestal* that correspond with her head, womb, and feet, respectively.

The third principle is that the elements of **air, fire, earth,** and **water** form the basic building blocks of any *Divine SelfQare Strategy*. The more elements you can strategically incorporate into each healing and wellness routine, the more effective the treatment and, in many cases, the results. But more on that later.

As far as Denkenesh is concerned, these *trans-physical* practices that involved the four elements were common to scores of women who both observed and maintained their bodies as sacred temples.

A Beautiful & Wonderful Sacred Temple

My loving grandchildren, if you are reading this right now, always remember that you are beautifully and wonderfully made to fulfill a Divine Purpose. You were carefully crafted in your mother's womb by the Most High who gave you a body designed to serve as a sacred temple. A temple holds great significance in the Kingdom of the Most High which is a Kingdom of Divine Light. It represents the awesome creative power of the All-Knowing One and it, therefore, houses all that which is sacred and right. This means you were born into royalty, and you are *royal*.

Also note, every *royal* temple has a *crown, throne,* and *pedestal* denoting the presence of royalty. What is interesting is that each of these royal symbols correspond with a part of the human body designed to facilitate one or more of the natural elements – particularly the sensory organs. I will explain how shortly. For now, just note each of the organs and elements listed below:

- **Eye** *corresponds to the **fire** element*
- **Mouth** *corresponds to the **water** element*
- **Ear** *corresponds to the **earth** element*
- **Nose** *corresponds to the **air** element*
- **Womb** *corresponds to all four elements of **air, fire, earth** and **water***
- **Feet** *correspond to the **earth** and **water** elements*

My sacred granddaughters, I want each of you to have an awareness of your body. Learn the basics that I will share with you here, but also study to prove your knowledge and wisdom about some basic functions of important parts of you, at both a physical and *trans-physical* level. We'll start with the organs that allow our bodies to experience and interpret the phenomena that occur in the external world.

As *Divine SelfQare* practitioners, and daughters of the Most High, we need to be aware of the functions of these organs and their importance. In other words, we need clear eyesight to *see* objects and activities as they take shape or happen within our environment. Yet, we have Divine Vision to interpret these events and things properly. We need clear hearing to hear sounds as they occur. In fact, we are designed to hear danger prior to seeing it, but it is Divine Listening that enables us to actively perceive and listen to the voice of the Creator. Similarly, clear speech is vital to effective communication. Yet Divine Speak facilitates ministry in the kind of tongue that can transform the world in a positive, lasting way while also transcending time, space and circumstances. Now that just pertains to the crown or head.

When it comes to the womb, (although I am referring to the entire female reproductive system right now, we will address the actual meaning of the word later) we are speaking to two aspects of being in the world. By this I mean, the process of physical creation, which is a science, and the process of Divine Creativity which is an art.

You see, my daughters and sons, the Most High placed a great deal of power and humanity in women by giving them wombs from which to birth physical life or humanity and perpetuate mental life, also known as ideas, or the humanities. So, a wise man will confide in his wife and supportive partner all that he aspires to achieve in his life. Subconsciously he is asking her to nurture his ideas in her spiritual womb. He is inviting her to help bring them to life (delivery). If she is in agreement with him, she will use her gifts to nurture his ideas by supporting him (gestation) and together, they utilize each other's creative resources to give those ideas a new form (life). This might take on the shape of an invention, a solution to a devastating problem, a cure for a disease, a book, a movie, or even a strategy for war. He, in essence, impregnates her (conception) at a subconscious or even spiritual level. Most wise and successful men of the Most High use this method to achieve their divine goals.

But, figuratively speaking, we as women do not need men to *'inseminate'* us with divine ideas. We are born with this independent power, and it is sourced directly from the Most High, enabling us to 'self-impregnate' ourselves using our innate gift of creative ingenuity and divine resourcefulness. I am living proof of this, I have given physical birth to a human being through the act of procreation with a man, and I have given spiritual birth to Divine Ideas with the help of the Most High using Divine Creativity. This book, for instance, is one example. Ironically, it took me very close to nine months to write and publish it. But this was only after three months of forming a visual concept of it in my mind first.

Once a great spiritual guide taught me that it actually takes one full year to create a baby; that conception begins in the spiritual realm - three months prior to the father and mother coming together for the act of Divine Procreation.

Irrespective of the criticism, this concept is likely to provoke among my learned readers. I was so moved by the idea that I modeled this in my personal life. Your father, Zakur, is an on-purpose child. I requested that he be here. I took steps to ensure he'd make it here. I will always be grateful to the Most High for facilitating and creating his life through me. My prayer is that one day he will be a dad.

Wherever this concept falls along the broad spectrum of your current belief system, be it full faith and credit, or unrealistic and impossible, I think it's an idea worthy of consideration as it is suggestive of heavenly influence into earthly matters - a thought that fascinates and inspires me. How about you?

Now, beloved, the pages to come will take you on a path that will help you explore the sacred temple we just talked about. The temple is a metaphor for how your body will become a guide as you learn more about the *crown, throne, pedestal*, and everything in between.

A Guide To The Body As A Sacred Temple

My sacred granddaughters and sons, I aspire to tell you about all the pertinent facts that pertain to each of the following body parts, but to also hold a comprehensive discussion related to them. These discussions and discoveries will help you create a holistic perspective of the main themes that I want to build upon. Read along, sacred grandchildren.

Crown | Head

Let's focus first on the eyes.

We'll start with making a distinction between basic eyesight and a heightened form of seeing that I refer to as Divine Vision.

Eyesight enables us to look at things around us, but vision, from a *trans-physical* perspective, allows us to perceive that which is beyond what our physical eyes can see. Perception, on the other hand, is more of an intellectual exercise and is an important aspect of planning and strategizing. This exercise enables us to bring something new into existence. Vision, therefore, is seeing the future before it comes into being, and this one special ability is what distinguishes human beings from all other animals. The latter may be able to see with physical eyes, sometimes better than humans; but they lack spiritual eyesight. Eagles for instance, have 20/4 sight. They even have the ability to see through ultraviolet light; but they are like all other creatures in the animal kingdom in their inability to formulate a vision of the desired future.

That is because this requires spiritual eyesight or Divine Vision. Even children, with their vivid imaginations, can visualize their future selves with a career as a doctor or anything else they want to be. With maturity, a child may map out a plan to achieve that goal. A sweet, young panda, however, is incapable of planning its way out of the national zoo and back to its natural habitat - one conducive for adult pandas. Spiritual eyesight, therefore, or Divine Vision is a very precious gift to humanity from the Most High, possessed by both men and women.

With Divine Vision comes the exercise and execution of will. How we see ourselves in relation to the future is important because it determines how and why we live out our lives. For instance, I have devoted a great deal of my life and some of my time to writing this book. I did so because I have vision. Vision tends to drive our activities in life and inspire us to look after the interests of others - not just our own. It also entails realizing that we are all connected and that your personal welfare and health are an extension of my own.

Back to the eyes...

Our eyes are capable of distinguishing between nearly 10 million different colors. Some have even said that the eyes are the lamps of the body. A lamp is a light source that also gives off heat - both of which correspond with *fire*, one of the four elements. Interestingly enough, the eye can cure itself of infection with the proper use of heat (but more on that later).

Mechanically speaking, the eyes function like a camera taking photos of our environment and sending those photos to the brain for processing or interpreting. Once transferred through a complex system of optical nerves, the brain begins to interpret these images using human experience, knowledge, culture, and values as a measuring tool. No pun intended, but doesn't this make *sense*?

Scientifically speaking, the human eye has proven to be a delicate, yet complex sensory organ that consists of an inner, middle, and outer membrane. The outer membrane is what is called 'the white' of the eye, but the part of the eye that functions as the 'camera' with its ability to refract light and remain transparent is the crystalline lens. The fastest muscles in your body are the ones that make the eyes blink. These muscles contract in less than a 100th of a second. In just one day, we may blink over 11,500 times.

Ancient Cosmetics Were Medicinal

Eyes are naturally protected by eyelashes which serve to keep minor irritants out of the eyes, such as dust, debris, sand, or dirt. But did you know that in ancient times (and even today) both men and women wore a special form of eyeliner called "*kohl*" or "*kuhl*" in Arabic to protect their eyes from environmental conditions like glaring sunlight rays, sand dust storms, and other harsh conditions?

Many falsely believe that when ancient people - particularly among Nile Valley civilization - are depicted in various art forms with thick black substance smeared around their eyes that they were merely expressing a unique type of cosmetic beauty. In actuality, many people were prone to eye diseases due to the harsh environmental conditions they lived in which are characteristic of many eastern regions to this day. Places in regions of North Africa, and places close to it are still subject to harsh weather like sand and dust storms, glaring sunlight, excessive heat, and flies that harm the health of the eyes.

This is due to the fact that the ancients mastered a recipe based on lead derivatives that were known to trigger an immunological response by seeping into the eye and actually preventing or reducing the incidence of blindness, cataracts, ocular scarring and other common infections that many still suffer from today, like conjunctivitis and sties. If you think that is questionable, consider the fact that scientists of recent times have discovered that the eyes are full of the type of bacteria shown to elicit an immune system response that prevents the growth of pathogens in the eye and keeps microbes under control as well.

Present Day Cosmetics Contrast With Divine SelfQare

The wisdom and Divine Healing traditions of ancient times have been usurped in modern times by corporate opportunism coupled with a quest for human perfection, popularly known by the term 'flawless look.' Together these two forces have unwittingly created a 532 billion dollar cosmetic industry, much of which I believe is harmful and counterproductive in a myriad of ways. They have resulted in infection, allergic reaction, irritation, and the loss of natural lashes, but worse, they can trap dirt and introduce new bacterial or fungal infections. Yet, according to the latest market trends reports, the eyelash industry is slated to reach 1.5 billion dollars in sales between 2019 and 2024. Similarly, top statistical reports highlight that 80% of the top ten brands in false eyelashes and adhesives belong to just two companies in the overall beauty industry.

Take for instance, false eyelash strips and eyelash extensions, a form of cosmetic applied to the eyelid to create feminine allure by giving women the appearance of having natural, thick, long, curly eyelashes. These lashes, made from human hair, animal fur, or synthetic fibers that simulate them, are problematic by themself; but the real danger to the eyes rests in the glue used to apply them. False extension glues often contain formaldehyde which at room temperature is a colorless, flammable gas with a very strong odor.

Formaldehyde is extremely irritating to the skin and yes, studies have shown formaldehyde and other ingredients found in biological glues can cause cancer. Even though people may come into contact with formaldehyde, being that it is a product of combustion, and can be found in many things like a gas stove and kerosene heater emissions, as well as, cigarette smoke, high rates of exposure pose a greater cancer threat - a risk that needs to be avoided at all costs.

Also consider how formaldehyde is the key ingredient used to formulate embalming fluid. Embalming fluid is a preserving liquid that delays decomposition. It is made up of 35% formaldehyde and is so dangerous that when being administered to the dead, no one is allowed to be in the room other than the embalmer. Formaldehyde was once used to anesthetize people for minor surgery. In fact, embalmers reduce the likelihood of being anesthetized by wearing personal protective equipment or PPE when working on the deceased.

According to several reports, makeup, shampoo, skin lotion, nail polish, and other personal care products contain chemical ingredients that lack safety data. Moreover, some of these chemicals have been linked in animal studies to male genital birth defects, decreased sperm counts, and altered pregnancy outcomes in women. My sacred granddaughters imagine the consequences of using these kinds of cosmetics peddled to the masses in a scheme that prioritizes profits over people.

Please realize, the FDA does not prevent cosmetic manufacturers from using formaldehyde in beauty industry products like eyelash glue. You do know what this means, right? Yes, every day, potentially millions of unsuspecting women and girls are exposing themselves to danger unnecessarily. But not you, I pray. Take heed of your Grandmother's wisdom and sustain your natural gift of Divine Vision and clear eyesight at all costs. *You are beauty.*

Natural Is Best - Beware Of Misleading Labels and Claims

There is a saying that moderation is everything and in many instances this is true. You should strive to avoid excessiveness and impulsivity in all areas of life generally, but especially when expressing your unique personality through physical beauty. I don't mean for you to avoid adorning beautiful colors to enhance your body or face. But I do want to warn you about making the mistake of trusting the labels found on beauty products claiming to be "natural" or even "organic" cosmetics. Unfortunately, these words may only refer to *specific* ingredients that may be certified organic, not all of the ingredients that the product holds.

Avoid cosmetic products that contain ethanolamine as they are often contaminated with cancer causing chemicals. Neither cosmetic products nor treatments require FDA approval, meaning perfumes, makeup, moisturizers, shampoos, hair dyes, face and body cleansers, and shaving products can end up on market shelves without any testing. Beware, sacred daughters, in today's world, *"words sell."* Commercial interests will simply assuage the fears of conscientious buyers with sweet words of comfort like 'home-made,' 'chemical-free,' or 'earth-friendly,'"when the truth is they may be sourcing these products from China and other countries where all manner of harmful chemicals may be used in the mass production of these cosmetics.

Exercise Creative Ingenuity

So, what is the solution? Creativity, knowledge, and the application of them both through wisdom. You must possess a natural inquisitiveness or innate desire to know things in life. Knowing how to create and produce that which is needed and desired is what empowered the health and freedom movements of our ancestors, and it will also sustain you.

There is nothing wrong with wanting to be as beautiful as you can. In fact, I encourage you to, but do so naturally with full consideration for the world we share with plants, animals and humanity. Take what you need but restore and replenish the earth as you do so. Start all beauty regimens by taking proper care of your body, mind, and spirit - especially while you're young. Begin with exercise, then practice proper hydration - nature's most effective moisturizer, by the way, is water, and of course, nutrition. You can also explore jewelry making with elements that reflect the beauty of the earth like copper, bamboo, turquoise, stones, and jewels.

Learn ways to make natural eyeliner, mascara, and natural lip tones using plants and even food. For instance, Have you ever noticed how cherry juice stains your fingertips? Well, they can also stain your lips on a lovely summer day as an organic, temporary lip color that can be topped with a tiny bit of coconut oil for a touch of shine! The possibilities are limitless, safe, clever and better yet, affordable!

Speaking of lips, let's turn now to the mouth...

Open your mouth and try to breathe in through it. You should discover that it doesn't feel natural. Mouth breathing has a lot of adverse effects that cause problems to the brain, facial structure, and bloodstream. Why? Because breathing is not a natural function of the mouth - that's what the nose is meant to do. But, if the nose is obstructed by something and can't pass air to your lungs, your mouth can assist temporarily.

So, what purpose then does our mouth serve? Good question! There are many important functions for the mouth, speech being just one of them. Remember when I said that clear speaking is vital to effective communication? I also stated that the Divine Oratory or Speak is what enables us to impact the world in a lasting, positive way.

What is the purpose of the mouth as a sensory organ?

Aside from speaking, and providing an alternative form of breathing, the mouth serves four other important functions; namely, masticating, tasting, structural appearance, and communicating through expression.

The different parts of the mouth enable these core functions. When we say mouth, we are collectively speaking of lips, jaw, tongue, teeth, floor, saliva, salivary glands, cheeks, palate and muscles.

I have provided some unique facts that tell us something interesting about each part below.

Lips - Lips help manage saliva and food inside the mouth. They move the food in between the teeth while we chew. They represent feelings of expression by smiling or frowning and convey words through speaking.

Jaw - The bone structure that holds the 32 human teeth in place.

Tongue - The tongue is an important muscle that aids in digestion by moving food around the mouth in preparation for mastication.

Teeth - Teeth are bone organs embedded in the mouth's upper and lower jaws and they are critical to the digestive system. They are for tearing and chewing food into pieces and they also help us with speech and sound formation.

Floor - The floor of the mouth, the portion of the mouth that rests beneath the tongue, made of mucous membranes covering the area from the lower jawbone gums back to the base of the tongue.

Saliva - Water accounts for 99.5 percent of the saliva in your mouth. The rest consists of enzymes, antibodies, and important proteins that aid in digestion, moistens food, and keeps the mouth clean.

Salivary Glands - Salivary glands produce saliva through major glands that rest on both sides of the mouth, but smaller glands are located in the cheeks, lips, oral cavity, tongue, and along the floor of the mouth.

Cheeks - The connective tissue, subcutaneous fat, and certain muscles form our cheeks. This important wall of the mouth is situated in the face area below the eyes to the lips, nestled between the nose and ears, along the front of the face to the lips. Interestingly, the same skin cells that make up a human vagina are the ones found in a human mouth.

Palate - The palate is what separates the mouth from the nasal cavity.

Mouth Muscles - Did you know that the strongest muscle in the human body is the masseter or the jaw muscle?

The mouth is intriguing in many ways and should not be taken for granted. But before you go kissing, be careful to note there are more bacteria in a human mouth than there are people in the world. A clean mouth is in the best position to resist bacterial infections. *Cleanliness is next to Godliness.* Hygiene is key.

Now, let's tune into a discussion about ears...

Our ears are powerful sensory organs that help us experience the world through sound. They facilitate the audible aspect of communication and connect us to life as it takes shape all around us through energetic vibration. Arguably, next to the gift of eyesight, hearing is next in importance. And since the planet is teeming with movement and sound vibrations, the ear organ corresponds to the earth.

A fact that never occurred to me before now is that the first three letters of the word earth are 'ear.' While this irony is pure coincidence - the two words don't appear to be derived from the same etymological origins - I can't help but notice the little nudges of support and encouragement I receive from the Most High. They feel like gifts of insight and hints that we are on the right path in our train of thought. It is as if the Most High is urging us to move forward with new or different ideas.

My sacred grandchildren, you must listen to me closely, as I talk about the art of spiritual hearing or Divine Listening. But before I do, I want to share some basic thoughts you may not know about sound, frequency, and vibration as they relate to hearing.

Every day our ears are inundated with noise. The sound, whether uplifting music from the radio, or the hum of a microwave oven, stems from movements back and forth that create sound waves. These sound waves travel through the air, but they can also travel through water and solid objects. Once these sound waves make it to our ears, however, they cause the eardrum to vibrate. When this happens, our brain interprets the sound and gives it meaning.

As humans, we typically hear a range of sounds measuring between 20 to 20,000 hertz. Anything below or above this is out of hearing range for most people. Consequently, we are deaf to many of the sounds other animals can sense through hearing. Yet so much of what we can't hear still affects us physically, spiritually, emotionally and in so many other ways.

Take for instance, that the earth vibrates, which means it makes a sound. The humming sound the earth makes when it vibrates is inaudible to us because it happens at such a low frequency. Danger is something heard before seen. This is especially true for animals. According to wildlife experts, earth vibrations, like those that lead to tsunamis, can be sensed by animals with their more acute hearing long before we get an idea of what's going on beneath the earth. The vibrations happening around us can affect our lives in good and bad ways whether we hear it or not. The key to surviving the dangers that we cannot detect with our natural hearing, may be heard through a different gift known as Divine Listening or hearing with our spiritual ear.

Divine Listening vs. Natural Hearing

The difference between our ability to hear in the natural world versus the spiritual realm which is the realm of the unseen is directly linked to actively listening in silence for the Divine One, the Most High, to speak to us about the world as it exists. Divine Listening is the active skill honed through the combined art of prayer, fasting, and meditation. When someone opens the line of communication to petition the Most High through prayer, they speak for a period of time in ways that either request help or acknowledge help already received. It is a one-sided conversation. Therefore, it could be said that prayer is the art of talking without listening.

But the opposite is true for meditation, which is the art of listening without speaking. The meditator actively disciplines the mind to listen for the subtle impression that comes from the Divine One, the Most High. Being skillful in both arts is a prerequisite to becoming an effective practitioner of *Divine SelfQare*.

Fasting, however, is an art that bears many fruits necessary to feed the soul. It literally and figuratively is the soul food of all humanity. Fasting is the concise art of abstaining to eliminate distractions that prevent us from fulfilling our life purpose or achieving a goal in alignment with that overall purpose. I have fasted for many periods over the course of developing and writing the concepts within this book for you to read at a given time if we are blessed. I fasted from food. Food is the most common distraction in life, but there are plenty of others. When we master the art of abstaining and couple this discipline with the art of prayer and meditation, we receive many gifts. The most precious of these is the gift of Divine Listening or Hearing that develops as we use our ears spiritually, giving us unobstructed access to the Divine One, the Most High.

A Lesson Worth Listening To...

I want to share the story of a wise grandmother whose skill in Divine Listening actually saved her life and the lives of her three grandchildren.

The story took place at a time in recent history when life was a lot less technological. There were no battery-operated smoke detectors to provide advance notice of a deadly fire, or indoor fire extinguishers. You couldn't just pick up a phone, dial 911 and expect a well-equipped fire department to aid you in a rescue. No, this was a simpler time, in the deep south. In a world shared between an aging but wise grandmother and her completely defenseless grandchildren who relied on her for everything at this point in time. Listen carefully beloved...

Ms. Hudson was traveling home from church with her grandchildren after a late Sunday service that went into the night. A kind couple from town agreed to drop them off since Ms. Hudson did not have a car. When they arrived home, she got out of the car and prepared to take her grandchildren and their belongings into the house. Instead, Ms. Hudson stood still and silently gazed indirectly towards the front door.

People were polite back then, so no one interrupted her for a few moments, but after a short while, the grandchildren began to ask questions and pull at her hand until she said "Shhh." The man driving observed the request and remained quiet until a bit more time passed with no change in Ms. Hudson's behavior. The wife of the driver was more attuned to the strange behavior, sensing that something important was taking place and that Ms. Hudson would soon come back from her silent meditation and inform them of what was happening. Ms. Hudson just continued staring off toward the door with her head positioned as if she were listening intently.

After a while, she said a prayer then quickly turned around and said to the driver and his wife, "We can't stay here tonight. Please take us to spend the night somewhere else. Somewhere away from here." She then inquired as to whether the driver and his wife would allow them to spend the night in their home. They agreed. The next day, they learned the house that Ms. Hudson owned, burned down to the ground the previous night - the night she refused to go inside with her grandchildren.

Listen To The First Voice

I am not surprised if you are wondering about the incident I just described. When I first heard it, I had two probing questions:

What did the grandmother know that night about the house?

And more importantly, *how did she know?*

Ms. Hudson seemed to know that she and her grandchildren were at risk of danger if they stayed in their own house that night. She knew because she obeyed what is referred to as 'the first voice' or the voice of the Divine Protector, The Most High.

Let me explain, during the period that she appeared to be transfixed on the house; she was actually receiving Divine Guidance from the Most High. This took the form of an inaudible sound that can only be heard by using the spiritual ear or the gift of Divine Listening. In scientific terms, what the grandmother 'heard' was outside the range of twenty 20 - 20,000 Hertz, which is the normal range of human hearing.

Not surprisingly, the information she received was so compelling that she felt compelled to contend with it in silence. As she stood there weighing the consequences of not being obedient, she appeared to be transfixed to onlookers, but she was really engaged in active or Divine Listening with her gift of spiritual hearing. But it is also possible that she came into contact with data so shocking that it forced her to wrestle over conflicting data that began to arise when she failed to act with immediacy on the instruction of the first voice.

I wonder how many innocent women, men, girls and boys have lost their precious lives to someone with wicked intentions simply because they ignored this very powerful first voice? It is so subtle that if you are not attuned to it, you could easily dismiss it. You might think it's just a fleeting thought or insecurity and not act on what is likely to be some critical information in the form of a warning, advice, instruction, urging, or even encouragement.

Oftentimes, people report getting 'a hunch' about someone or something. They get clear guidance about a course of action to take. Yet, they fail to act on the first voice, oftentimes, to their own detriment. The longer a person delays acting on the advice and counsel of the first voice, the greater the chance they will begin to wrestle over seemingly conflicting guidance, doubting whether what they 'heard' in the first instance was sound information (no pun intended).

Beloved, always remember that when we doubt the guidance, we receive from the Most High which was intended for us we will start to receive conflicting information. This conflicting information is usually the voice of the enemy who is also known as the wicked one.

For instance, a person might be instructed to steer right at a traffic intersection and follow that guidance only to find out later that they avoided a potentially bad traffic accident just a mile ahead that would have cost them two hours of important travel time. Similarly, one might be instructed to go back inside the house before pulling off in their car but ignore this instruction only to find out that they left an important document at home that was needed to file a claim in court and consequently missed an important deadline in a critical legal case.

The difference between the two outcomes stems from not acting immediately on the instruction of the first voice which would have assisted them with something they needed or should have been aware of. Instead, the second person got caught up in the spiritual tug of war that happens when Divine Guidance is received but not acted on immediately, allowing a second or dissenting voice to enter and introduce doubt, providing conflicting advice that literally causes an internal debate over a particular course of action. Avoid this. Act on the first voice.

Developing your spiritual ear to master the art of Divine Listening today is vitally important. It saves lives.

Have you ever heard people talk about events they didn't attend? Or places they went to during various periods in their lives that are forever marked in their memories because these were times that they believe they avoided an injury or could have died but for "*something*" telling them not to go to a specific place as planned? They later found out that their obedience to that guidance saved them pain, money, or even their lives due to missing out on a potentially negative event that took place in that very location they were going to at the exact time they were scheduled to be there. This happens quite often.

Sometimes the opposite is true and following the first voice leads to happiness. For instance, people sometimes report good things happening as a consequence of following guidance 'heard' in the spiritual ear. Like 'accidentally' discovering that they left their house keys in the door. When they return home to recover something else, they instead recover their keys from the door so grateful that no one could enter the house undetected! This gift happened as a consequence of being obedient to the first voice.

This phenomenon is known as the *first voice* to us as Daughters of the Most High and it is Divine Guidance from the source of all life as the Great Protector. The sound of Divine Guidance can't always be heard with your physical ear because it is a frequency so unusual that it is often felt or experienced by those with a heightened sense of spiritual awareness.

The key takeaway from this is that we are currently living in a time when people have no sense of spiritual hearing to warn them of life's pitfalls and traps, so they fall victim to a number of cunning strategies. Listen to me, sacred granddaughters and sons; with your spiritual ear you can hear danger long before you see it. But it is important for you to hone spiritual hearing or *Divine Listening* skills well enough to develop and use this gift of knowing.

A Note On Your Nose

Your nose does more than just decorate your face. Inside, you're carrying around a personal air treatment system, cleverly designed to protect the delicate tissues of your lungs that transfer oxygen out of the air you breathe and into your body.

Our nose is one of the most complex sensory organs. It is instrumental in keeping you safe, sensual, and sensitive to changes in your environment. As the first organ in the respiratory system, it functions to humidify the air you breathe, and most importantly it facilitates breathing.

It is responsible for helping to process the sound of your voice. The nose can trigger good or bad memories so be mindful to keep attractive, clean smells available in your home, work, and social environments.

Although you can't always control the temperature or contents of the air you breathe, you can take steps to keep your nose as healthy as possible by drinking plenty of water to keep mucus thin and fluid, helping warm the air you breathe in cold weather by wearing a scarf over your nose and mouth or keeping nasal passages moist by gently inhaling soothing, therapeutic grade essential oils like peppermint and eucalyptus, especially if you are exposed to dry air, allergens or have an infection. You can and should also keep green, detoxifying plants in your home environment to help purify the air you breathe.

As we've now touched upon each crevice of the crown, going into the depth of everything, it's time to mount upon the knowledge of your sacred throne. The pages to come will shed light on the significance of a womb, both biologically and *trans-physically*.

Throne | Womb

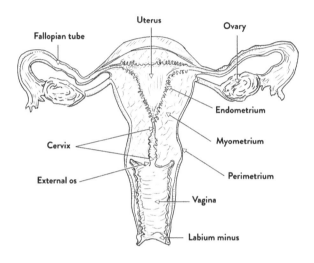

Over the course of writing this book, I have used the term *womb* generally to mean the entire creative center and female reproductive system. However, you should know the medical definition of the womb differs significantly from the *trans-physical* meaning that I have used thus far. As your grandmother and matriarch, I have a duty to clarify what I mean, and give you an accurate depiction of the realities of womanhood. In addition, I want you to be able to intelligently and accurately articulate your needs as a woman whenever you may feel the need to do so with your doctor, spouse, or as a *Divine SelfQare* practitioner helping yourself and other women. But, in order to do this accurately requires familiarity with the medical definitions of our key reproductive organs and their functions. What I am about to share with you is not exhaustive but it's a decent start and points you in the right direction as you continue to develop knowledge and wisdom about the human body and its reproductive power as a woman.

The female body is not only beautiful, but also well-designed and highly suited to procreate, nurture, and sustain the life of humanity. This is why, I will make an effort to explain to you how the key parts of your female organs work in the following segment starting with understanding the womb and other parts of the reproductive system including the uterus, ovaries, fallopian tubes, cervix, cervical opening, vagina, vaginal opening, and vulva.

When a woman is blessed with a child, her belly expands to accommodate the new life. The organ that is responsible for housing this new life or baby, as well as the umbilical cord and placenta is known medically as the womb. It is larger than the uterus because it is constantly expanding to meet the needs of the growing baby. And, if all goes well, the baby, umbilical cord and placenta, remain safely in the womb for the entire gestation period. Therefore, we can affirm that the womb is absolutely vital to life as a powerful component of the procreative process.

Trans-physically speaking, a woman can be pregnant with ideas, solutions, and dreams of a higher life. When she is, her ideological womb is activated as her body flows with creative ingenuity or Divine Creativity! Thus, when you hear me speak of the womb in this sense, know that I am collectively referring to the medical and spiritual definition of a woman's womb as the *creative* center for life, since a woman with a fertile mind and a heart that nurtures is full of life and birth potential as well.

But let's get back to the rest of the female reproductive organs...

You should know something about this particular aspect of a woman's life that causes a great deal of anxiety for women - the menstrual cycle or period. My prayer is that you will also find joy in having a healthy, painless period. There are many things that can facilitate this including regular exercise, a healthy vegan diet, and plenty of alkaline, pure, mineral-rich water that helps to alkalize your blood. Your menstrual cycle is an important part of your life as a woman. Embrace and understand how it plays a pivotal role in your reproductive health as a woman and potentially as a mother.

In the course of her life, an average woman will experience a period or menstruation for about 40 years. Menstruation is bleeding on a monthly basis in order to discard the build-up that forms from the endometrium at the time of ovulation. Ovulation is your body's way of preparing for the conception of life or the fertilization of an egg. When the egg isn't fertilized, the endometrium layer sheds, and this is what we refer to as your period.

The menstruation or blood flows from your uterus through an opening in your cervix, then passes down your vaginal canal and out of the vaginal opening. We prevent this blood from staining our clothes by wearing a non-toxic, reusable cloth that sometimes contains activated charcoal called a menstrual pad during our monthly menstrual cycle. We can safely wear these pads with confidence. Then they are washed thoroughly by hand and/or machine to protect our bodies from harsh chemicals that interrupt the delicate balance of hormones within our bodies. Doing this also shows a great deal of responsible concern and consideration for the environment. Reusable pads are hygienic and reduce the tons of biological waste that disposal pads and tampons contribute to the overburdening of the environment.

The uterus is the organ responsible for producing our menstrual cycle each month. It is a hollow, pear shaped organ that rests behind the bladder within the pelvic cavity. More importantly, it is the main reproductive organ we have as women. The three layers of tissue and muscles that make up our uterus play a vital role in our reproductive health and fertility. These layers are the *endometrium* or inner layer, the *myometrium* or middle layer, and the *perimetrium* or outer layer. When an egg is fertilized it makes its way into the inner layer of the uterus or the endometrium and implants itself. But fertilization itself usually takes place in the fallopian tubes.

Fallopian tubes serve as the bridge between the ovaries and the uterus. The ovaries house the ovum or eggs. Beloved, did you know that a woman is born with all the eggs she will ever have right inside of her ovaries? If you think about it, you will come to realize something miraculous. Aside from the fact that our bodies hold an estimated seven million eggs at the time of birth, the eggs you are carrying right now were once inside your mother when you were a fetus in her womb, your eggs were there inside her too! If that doesn't blow your mind, this also means that your eggs were once inside your grandmother because when she carried your mother, your mother was a fetus who was carrying the egg or ovum that became you. Now doesn't this fact give added meaning to the connection we share with our predecessor matriarchs? We literally existed inside our grandmother as an unfertilized egg for a period of time. Life is miraculous and astounding!

Before we conclude our womb discussion, let's cover a few more things...

Women sometimes use the term vagina when speaking about the flesh that forms the external portion of the female genitalia. While this is very close, it's not exactly right, anatomically speaking. When you stand in front of a mirror naked, the part of your female reproductive system that you can see is called the *vulva*. This term refers collectively to the flesh or skin you can see and everything inside your outer lips also known as the *outer labia* or *labia majora*. The parts you find inside the outer lips include the inner lips or *labia minora*, the vestibule or the innermost part of the vulva, the urethral opening from which urination is expelled, the *clitoris*, and the *clitoral opening*. Now, what we think of as the *vagina* is actually the *vaginal opening*. This opening leads to the vagina, which consists of inner walls. These walls can expand to form a tubular canal but stick together when in a relaxed state.

Despite the diagrams you'll encounter in textbooks or the internet that depict the vagina as a long smooth tube, you must understand that this is not factual. In reality, the vagina has these internal *clitoral bulbs* at the base or bottom, located on either side. In addition, there is a deep aspect of the vagina, which is located close to the *cervix*. Both the bottom of the vagina and the deep vagina contain lots of nerves responsible for the pain or pleasure a woman can feel during sexual intercourse depending on her state of arousal. What I mean here is that when a woman is sufficiently aroused prior to sexual intercourse, the experience can be one of pure pleasure for her. This is because the upper two-thirds of her vagina stretches enough to allow for easier and deeper penetration by the male's reproductive organ or his penis without causing vaginal trauma as a result of injuring or bruising the cervix.

Remember that the uterus is the main organ of the reproductive system responsible for many aspects of a woman's health, pregnancy and sexual experiences. The cervix is the front part of the uterus. It has a small opening called the *external os* that enables menstrual blood to exit the uterus but also allows a baby to pass through into the vagina or birth canal.

In this manner, the womb is sacred as the creative center for life which aligns perfectly with your Divine Purpose. Therefore, you should honor this precious aspect of your being by being centered in your purpose through a *Divine SelfQare Strategy* that includes vaginal steaming. My granddaughters, we have already experienced vaginal smoking through the story of Denkenesh. But vaginal steaming is another powerful method of centering women in Divine Creativity and is also based on the ancient science of *trans-physics* by way of the four elements – **air, fire, earth** and **water**. This ancient science can help you unlock your hidden potential for creative ingenuity and divine healing.

Now that your head is elevated with a *crown* and your womb is centered on a *throne*, it's time to direct your attention to the *pedestal* - the foundation that supports your Sacred Temple.

Pedestal | Feet

Other than the head and the womb, our feet also play an incredibly essential role in our health. Do you remember the time I told you about how Grandmother Betty always urged me to put my feet up whenever I got the chance? Or to not walk on cold hard floors without slippers on? Our feet are like an entryway to the rest of our bodies. Many cultures believe the toes to be a pathway for bacteria to enter our body, which is why we tend to keep them covered from the harsh environment especially in colder seasons.

Feet are often overlooked when it comes to our health and wellbeing as women. My prayer and purpose in writing this part of the book are so that this will never be the kind of mistake that you will make. Your feet can play an instrumental role in your life, including helping you get to your goals. Please don't take them for granted. Yet, don't go to the other extreme by focusing all your time on making them meet today's beauty standards by focusing all your money and efforts on nail polish as opposed to good nail hygiene.

Pay special attention to the bottom of your feet and most importantly acknowledge any discomfort to your feet's bone structure. Avoid wearing tight, uncomfortable, or ill-fitted shoes. The price for neglecting your feet can be expensive in the long run, but the steps required to have healthy, strong, sturdy feet that can get you through life in its entirety are worth every cent. *The Divine SelfQare Strategy* and associated methods will save you thousands of dollars over time with your at-home spa treatments.

There are many ways people fail to honor the complexity of their feet, taking them for granted. This is partly because there are so many important things hidden in your feet. For instance, did you know that 25% of the bones in an adult human are located in the feet? With so many bones at risk each day, people who engage in a range of activities from jogging to dancing and other activities like working on your feet, or worse, being at risk of dropping heavy items on them in the course of work, are at risk of experiencing foot and ankle trauma. Unfortunately, many can attest to the fact that these types of injuries can lead to permanent disability or chronic pain - especially for those who don't seek proper treatment.

Let's take a look at some common but often misunderstood foot and ankle related injuries that can be avoided with proper care and attention:

Ankle Pain - It could be a sign of damage or injury to connective tissues, bones, muscles, or other components in your ankle joint.

Bunion - A bunion is a bone deformity that occurs when the joint at the base of your big toe becomes enlarged as your toe shifts out of place. Because bunions can cause chronic pain, stiffness, and swelling, they can be pretty uncomfortable to deal with.

Calluses (hyperkeratosis) - These are dry, flaky, hardened patches of skin that form because of constant friction over a bony area. If you have thickened calluses, *Divine SelfQare* foot soaks, and natural moisturizers are the answer.

Corns - These are small calluses that form on your toes because your tiny toe bones push up against your shoes and put pressure on your skin. These calluses are also notorious for causing pain and discomfort.

Hammertoes - This can lead to chronic toe pain and stiffness, as well as ongoing issues with corns.

Fungus Toenails (onychomycosis) - Fungus can cause your toenails to become so brittle and damaged, they may flake away or fall off over time.

Ingrown Toenails (onychocryptosis) - This may commonly lead to pain, redness, and inflammation. Since ingrown toenails can become seriously infected, it is wise to seek medical attention as soon as possible.

Neuroma - If it feels like your sock is always bunched up or that you regularly have a pebble in your shoe, even though everything is fine, chances are, you have a neuroma. If left untreated, neuromas can lead to chronic stabbing pain.

Plantar warts/Foot warts — These warts aren't just a nuisance, rather, they can cause pain and discomfort with each step you take.

Tendonitis - This means that you overstretched, overused, or even tore one or more of the tendons in your foot or ankle, which leads to inflammation.

My precious grandchildren, you must remember that throbbing, aching, swollen heels are often a sign of plantar fasciitis, injury, or even arthritis. If you suffer from heel pain on a daily basis, you should immediately resort to healing practices to relieve the pain. We will discuss more on healing practices for the pedestal in the next chapter of the book.

Treasures Of Sacred Knowledge

Now, my beloved daughters, it is time to relate to you how the healing practices of our wise ancestors, coupled with the sacred knowledge of *trans-physics*, inform us today as we journey in pursuit of our own Divine Health. You should recall that Divine Health means to be in excellent physical condition, to possess a sound mind, and to experience spiritual balance. And this, we should and can seek to do at any age. But stated another way, when our physical, mental, and spiritual bodies operate in Divine Order, this is called living in Total Body Alignment.

Thus, all the healing and wellness traditions I have shared through stories about our grand matriarchs; to those relayed about our collective ancestors from the period of bondage in this country; all the way back to a time when ancient Ethiopian women thrived in holistic health and womb wellness had an important contribution to make towards our individual journeys toward a state of Divine Health.

This would include, but not be limited to, four generations of women beyond me - namely, Grandmother Betty, Great-grandmother Lena Mae, and Great-great-grandmother Rebecca. It would encompass those resilient ancestors who preceded them, including the wise and honorable Frederick Douglas, QM Harriet Tubman, QM Harriet Jacobs, Reverend Dr. Martin Luther King, Elders Gus Smith and Sally Brown. And finally, culminate with the story of Denkenesh. When all of this wisdom is examined together - meaning those whose knowledge of *trans-physics* reveal a collective wealth of healing modalities - it is both frightening and intriguing to think of the progress in medicine and healing that could be possible today. If the chain of wisdom among the various healing traditions of African people remained unbroken for the last five centuries, what wonders and progress in health might have been? The need to address this question is partly what drives and inspires me to write this book.

The purpose of this book is much deeper than surface information about wellness strategies. It is to teach you how to employ and enjoy *trans-physics*. Recall that Dr. Martin Luther King Jr. revealed this great, but little-known science to the world on the night before his very assassination. It seemed as though he wanted to ensure that we were able to employ the same knowledge and wisdom that empowered many great people throughout history to protect themselves from death and disease or proclaim freedom from bondage.

Trans-physics is the weapon of the oppressed. It frees them from the oppression of the body, mind and spirit. It is a gift from the Most High and all of the civil rights and self-emancipation struggles of the past are replete with examples of *trans-physics* in action. In fact, history is full of skilled *trans-physicists* like QM Harriet Tubman who consistently employed the four elements along with her divine intentions to overcome obstacles in her way to health and freedom.

What she knew as a *trans-physicist* is that this can only be done with the fifth and most important element - the element of **Divine Intent**. **Divine Intent** represents the high ambition of humanity. It is always in alignment with the will of the Most High and is expressed aloud in the form of prayer, speeches, spirituality and petitions. When these are raised up to the Kingdom of Heaven, also known as the Kingdom of Light, powerful things happen for people who believe and have faith.

When it comes to personal health and wellness, the same science can be applied by you. That is why you will observe how the methods of *Divine SelfQare* expressed in this book are not typical self-care treatments by today's standards. They are so much more than what one can expect from a trip to a salon or sauna. It goes beyond the pedicures, manicures, nail extensions, and hair removal treatments that many of us are accustomed to, or the invasive suctioning of various body parts to produce specific outcomes. No, that is not the aim of *Divine SelfQare*.

Yes, beloved grandchildren, this treasure of knowledge that you now possess an awareness of, are instrumental to your understanding of the origins of *Divine SelfQare*. Our sacred method of pursuing overall body wellness and womb health is rooted in something special and divine. My precious children, if you are ready to take control of your health, wholeness, and longevity, these simple ideas will empower, strengthen and propel you to victory!

Remember, Daughters of the Most High, we aspire to use our bodies wisely; to treat our bodies respectfully; and to manage and protect the health and wellness of our bodies responsibly. This physical body is a gift from the Most High. It is what I refer to as our Queendom because its proper management involves a special set of skills, knowledge, and tools that I refer to as Queendom Qare.

We do this *Divine SelfQare* as a means of assuring that we are able to effectively fulfill our Divine Purpose as mothers, daughters of the Most High, wives, sisters, inventors, healers, teachers, business owners and creative innovators. But of equal importance, sacred daughters, is that you learn to enjoy your own bodies. Beloved, what I am stating here is that you too must appreciate your own body in all of its beauty, gifts, and capabilities.

Another way to conceptualize this is through the wisdom of the flight attendant. A flight attendant specifically instructs airplane passengers prior to taking off that in the event of an emergency we must not attempt to help anyone else until we have applied the life-giving oxygen mask to our own face first.

Now isn't this instruction full of wisdom, granddaughters? Truthfully, an empty can cannot replenish the oil of another.

What the story of Denkenesh was attempting to relay to you, my beautiful daughters, is that we as women not only deserve to pour into ourselves the time, healing, and attention that we need to thrive - but in all reality, we actually have to - and not just for our own sakes but for everyone who depends on us to operate optimally in order to create and nurture life.

Trust me, daughters; you need no one's permission to do this for yourself. But if it helps, and until you develop your courage, you may fall back on your Grandmother's wisdom admonishing you to do so until you have embodied the principles of *Divine SelfQare* as law for yourself. My sacred one, you must advocate fiercely and effectively for yourself - just like Denkenesh, for she is our ancient proto-type of *Divine SelfQare* and we can model her with all of her effortless communications to her husband, expressing herself about what she needed (*the time for wellness*); where she needed it (*near the veranda*); and when she needed it (*presently*). Divine Health is the Creator's will for you too. The Most High created you — body, mind, and spirit — with a desire to prosper you and for you to live a long life full of health while on earth.

I have learned from experience that when it comes to women and the myriad of expressions of womanhood, people in general and men in particular *do not* value a *martyr*. Don't fall for those men, who purport to admire the meekest, most unassuming, voiceless women publicly; but in their secret hearts strongly desire and even crave women who place a high value on themselves as expressed through their visual presentation, clear ambition and respect demanded through a healthy dose of self-love. In other words, by no means should you present yourself as homely, unkempt, and self-sacrificing to the point of unattractiveness on behalf of some false notion of humility in a religious sense or otherwise.

That being said, my daughters and sons, you must set boundaries accordingly. Pay attention to how people react to the boundaries you establish. The best people to surround yourselves with are the people who support you. Conversely, offer your support to people who are setting their own boundaries, and respect their boundaries as well. Improve yourself. Accept yourself, understand yourself, forgive yourself, inform yourself, and love yourself. This is the beginning of strong, healthy relationships with others. Show up with dignity, honor, and presence in all spaces.

Make anyone and everyone who wants to participate in your life and benefit from your creative ingenuity acknowledge and respect this one true boundary you are entitled to as a daughter of the Most High, and that is, your right to engage in *Divine SelfQare*. Remember, you are as singularly divine as the sons and daughters of the Most High. You are already complete. Let this be your daily motto:

> *"As a Daughter of the Most High, I honor my body, spirit, and mind. Any person who has the privilege of sharing my life, who is the beneficiary of my love, and with whom I share my time, whether I am fulfilling my life work as a wife, mother, sister, advisor, or friend, will have to respect my boundaries and need for Divine SelfQare."*
> *Thus, Sayeth You (and your wise Grandmother)*

Make this statement your affirmation or apart of your *Divine SelfQare manifesto* and embrace it as your own personal declaration of Divine Health.

In the *Divine SelfQare* Manifesto below, observe the affirmational statements. Each one will remind you of the obligation that you have to protect, preserve, and perpetuate your own wellness through *Divine SelfQare!*

The Divine Self2are Strategy

I am a daughter of the MOST HIGH

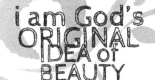

I HONOR AND PROTECT MY WOMB AS A SACRED SPACE FOR LIFE

I honor my body as a divine machine God loaned me to achieve my sacred purpose

I am patient, thoughtful, and kind to myself

I share useful information with my sisters   i honor my body as a gift from the creator

I honor the divine resilience, womanhood, and spirit of my ancestors

I AM A VESSEL FOR TRUTH, LOVE, SOLUTIONS AND RIGHT INFORMATION

i RECOGNIZE THAT i NEED TO BE IN A STATE OF DIVINE HEALTH TO BE MY ABSOLUTE BEST

● ●

I AM CREATIVE, INTELLIGENT, AND PIONEERING WHEN EXPERIENCING OPTIMAL HEALTH

I seek the wisdom of the women who embody the essence of divine womanhood

I DRINK WATER DAILY

I seek knowledge that will help sustain my health
I practice self-respect, self-care, and self-love
I pray, fast, & meditate to connect with the Most High
I study the healing power of herbs

I am the evidence of the faith and hope of my ancestors

i VALUE having Dominion over MY life AND the Discipline necessary To sustain IT

I strive to be an example of divine health and beauty to the Daughters of the Most High

I Will Walk, Dance, Jump, Stretch & Bend

I work daily to achieve a state of divine health naturally

I SECURE MY OWN PHYSICAL SPIRITUAL AND MENTAL WELL-BEING AND ENCOURAGE FUTURE GENERATIONS TO DO THE SAME

i master use of essential oils for beauty, valor, wisdom and healing

Create Your Personal Divine SelfQare Environment

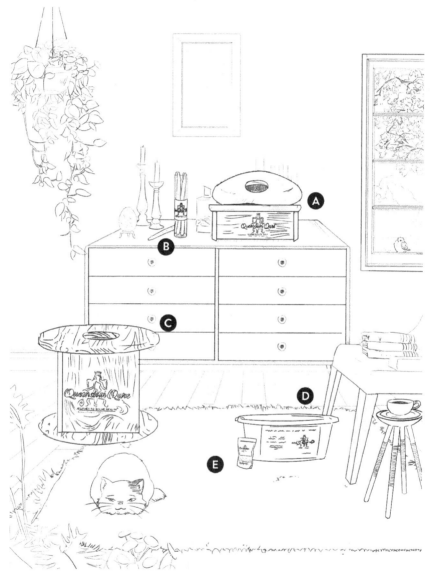

Key: A – Qrown Qare Steam Station. B – Ear Qones or Ear Qandles. C – Throne Qare Steam Station. D - Queendom Qare Foot Basin. E - Queendom Qare Foot Soak

My beloved granddaughters, now that you have a basic guide explaining the need for the cleansing of your body from your head to your feet, let's discuss how to create a safe and nurturing space in your home just as our example set by Denkenesh in creating her home wellness center in the quarters of her yard. Just as in ancient times, I want you to have an area in your home that enables you to focus on yourself without the distractions of the world interfering with your routine.

My beautiful granddaughters, you don't need to leave your home to introduce *Divine SelfQare* into your routine. As you deserve to have your own space, here is what I call the A, B. C's of creating a simple but satisfying at-home spa that you will cherish, enjoy and love.

Following the footsteps of Denkenesh, and keeping the above illustrated guide in mind, let's take a look at what you can do:

A. Assign a space in your home - *Choosing a sacred place*

Before you begin your journey to *Divine SelfQare,* my sacred granddaughters, it is important to select an area that makes you feel at ease and relaxed. Set up a sacred space in your home for the sole aim of promoting health and wellness. Depending on the space available, it might be a little nook in your bedroom or a larger area, as long as your objective is to create a space dedicated to your well-being. Remember how Denkenesh chose a place close to the juniper tree in her yard? Similarly, choose something that is special to you, something that soothes your mind and soul.

When you've found a peaceful sanctuary that nurtures your physical and mental health, it's critical that this wellness room or space be separated from distractions, clutter, and other reminders of worldly tasks so you can retreat there for the purpose of reinvigorating the mind as well as the body. The main goal is to achieve Total Body Alignment. Naturally, the space you choose plays an integral role.

B. Beautify the space with natural elements - *Elevating your sacred space*

You may start decorating your space now that you have one, and while you can set it up in any way you like, you should try to incorporate natural elements that inspire beauty while reflecting your awareness of the healing power of the four elements. Natural elements are very cleansing. Thus, use them for your own healing, preventative wellness treatments, and pure relaxation.

Having natural light in your at-home spa is an excellent approach to creating a relaxing atmosphere. This may be done with fragrant candles or a window to make the place feel brighter and more pleasant. Being out in the open, just like Denkenesh, can make the process feel much more natural, sensational, and relaxing. However, if you cannot access space under the sun, then you can make an inside space work just as well. Your comfort is always the priority, my sacred granddaughters.

You can also reap the benefits of aromatherapy by using a therapeutic blend of diverse aromas or independently such as ginger, tea tree, lavender, eucalyptus, peppermint, and other therapeutic-grade essential oils to eliminate impurities from inside, transforming your mood and productivity. Essential oils are a smart addition, but you can also go use plants like fresh eucalyptus, or flowers like lavender, baby's breath, and jasmine to clear, freshen and scent the air if you do not own a diffuser, or in addition to it if do you have one.

Indoor plants may also provide a lot of value in creating a healthy environment. These plants can improve your mental well-being while also being visually stimulating. Plants are as close as you can get to nature, and they can provide a sense of comfort, relaxation, and serenity, all of which are important in a wellness area.

There's so much you can do with your space by simply adding an oil diffuser, a small table, a gentle light, soft rug, or anything else that you think will help you create a peaceful space. The key is to remain uncluttered.

C. Crown your space with a throne - *Supporting your Feminine Essence*

Now that you've got the foundation in place, it's time to add the Divine Tools and equipment. This is when you should add your very own *Throne Qare Steam Station*. It's the most important feature of your at-home personal sacred wellness space. This is the ideal technique to practice the *Divine SelfQare* method of vaginal steaming anytime you choose.

Vaginal steaming, an ancient type of hydrotherapy, has been utilized by women across the African continent and other regions of the world for thousands of years. The purpose of this practice is similar to smoking or weybatis as we observed in the Denkenesh story, but steaming has been used in other places as well. For instance, women in various regions including Mozambique, Ghana, Nigeria, and South Africa, have employed the primary elements of **water** and **fire** to create steam for vaginal cleansing as opposed to **earth** and **fire** which create smoke. Both strategies are good, and they both employ the science of *trans-physics*. However, vaginal steaming is more conducive to the limitations of an indoor at-home spa and much safer.

The key thing to remember is that when you expose the womb to a specific herbal essence through a moderate form of heated air as either smoke or steam, it releases the essential oils from plants to create a sense of healing and well-being in these delicate regions of a woman's womb.

These herbs' potent therapeutic and healing properties are selected to expedite the process of healing from any vaginal injuries related to sexual intercourse, childbirth, hysterectomies, abortion, or the loss of virginity that a woman may sometimes experience over the course of her life. From the comfort of your own home, the specially designed *Throne Qare Steam Station* allows you to improve your health, cleanse, condition, and manage your sacred throne regions while honoring your womb and needs for relaxation and wellness.

Every Queen, in addition to a *Throne Qare Steam Station*, needs a flowing gown to wear while she steams. For a royal wellness experience, our *Throne Qare Steam Gown* and *Eye Qover* are must-haves. For mild vaginal steaming or womb wellness, the *Steam Gown* and *Eye Qover* are fashioned with a thick, soft, pure white cotton fabric.

Don't hold back my sacred granddaughters, and feel free to comfort yourself further with a *Plush Pillow* for the ultimate womb hydrotherapy experience. This addition to your personal *Throne* increases the comfort of your *SelfQare* moment. As you recover on your *Throne*, this cushion nestles nicely on top of your earthy, wood, hand-made steam station, allowing you to enjoy the soft, rich sensation of soft, plush, and comforting cotton.

Your *Throne* should not only be visually appealing, but you should also include an aromatic herbal blend that fills the air with a therapeutic essence that cleanses your space while having a positive effect on your health and wellness. Currently, the *Throne Qare Herbal Blends* provide a unique combination of herbs that can set you on your feminine wellness journey, but you can always research and develop your own blends to enhance your at-home spa, womb wellness experience.

D. Dedicate your space to the Divine - *Giving thanks to the Most High*

Your space is a sacred and dedicated area that is for the sole purpose of restoring and healing your physical and spiritual body. Embrace the journey that you aim to experience in your space and offer a prayer of gratitude to the Most High for your health and wellness. Don't forget to ask the creator for guidance, patience, intimacy, and intuition when praying so you can experience love, peace, and life from a Divine Perspective.

Having the strength to embrace your beauty comes from a Divine approach to health which can help you achieve physical, mental, and spiritual wellness. This is something that you can achieve by surrendering and seeking to align yourself with the Creator of all life through fasting, meditation, and prayer.

E. Establish a wellness routine - *Immersing yourself in Divine SelfQare*

Daughters of the Most High, the peace you attain by having a sense of direction and stability in your life are an incomparable feeling. If you're looking for some semblance of security, you'll need to establish a routine to practice *Divine SelfQare* methods. You're not creating a space so it can simply exist; you need to actually take the time to enjoy it.

Start by establishing a regular time for natural healing and wellness, so you can make the most of the luxurious experience to relieve yourself of stress through steaming. The long-term benefits can only be realized if you establish a wellness routine as a lifestyle deeply rooted in divinity to transform your emotional, physical, and spiritual well-being.

So, beloved, try to actively involve yourself in wellness as a part of the journey to Divine Health and take time out of your busy schedule to heal, rejuvenate, and pamper yourself with a *Divine SelfQare Strategy*, just like Denkenesh.

Chapter 9

Divine SelfQare Overview

Divine SelfQare is an approach to women's wellness that re-introduces ancient healing traditions which enabled women of the past to improve their health and achieve an overall sense of wellness using the tools of nature. In fact, the four elements were the building blocks of all-natural healing strategies and medicines. Whether it was harvested plants and tree bark for herbal remedies, or oils and salves to soothe away their pain and bruises. The men and women of the past not only employed a variety of approaches to enhance the sensual experiences of life through scent, sight, taste, and touch; but they relied on these tools to prevent disease and stave off death as well.

The Divine SelfQare Strategy is built on these foundational principles. While the methods we use to achieve *Total Body Alignment* in this day and age can be summed up as *Divine SelfQare*, the specific tools or assets that practitioners need to carry out these methods are collectively known as Queendom Qare assets specific to *Crown Qare, Throne Qare,* and *Pedestal Qare*.

Crown Qare products address the needs of the head. Throne Qare products focus on womb wellness activities; and Pedestal Qare products or assets address the feet. They can be acquired online via queendomqare.com.

Queendom Qare is a woman-owned company. Women handcraft the products with divine intent as expressed through divine prayer to the Most High. Blessings are a key ingredient in our products. They are what lead to a sense of Divine Wellness, femininity, and hygiene for our patrons. Women seek out Queendom Qare's line of quality products because they trust our work as a means of restoring emotional balance, rejuvenating the spirit, and promoting cellular rejuvenation.

At Queendom Qare, we focus on quality, health, and safety. You can expect to find pure essential oils, organic herbs, authentic designs, and untreated wood. Our *Throne Qare and Crown Qare Steam Stations* are not treated with chemicals, painted, or stained. Women can expect an earthy, clean, comfortable surface that is safe for direct skin contact when steaming on their Throne Qare (womb) or Crown Qare (head) Steam Stations.

The Divine SelfQare Strategy does not require you to compromise your health by exposing you to substances you can't possibly know the chemical composition of that have the potential to weaken your immune system. What makes *SelfQare Divine* is that it is meant to make you feel like a freshly watered garden, full, and teaming with life. It is meant to make you feel energized like a spring whose water never gets depleted. What is so beautiful is that in the process of doing so, the skin on your face will glow youthfully, your hearing will improve, your eyes will shine bright, your vision will get clearer, your mouth will feel and smell good, your womb will feel lighter and refreshed, and your feet will become softer, while giving you a better sense of stability.

The totality of all this is an elevated head, full of enlightenment and inspiration; a centered womb, full of creativity and fertile with divine ideas, and feet that are grounded and secure. In other words, *Total Body Alignment* has been achieved. The key is to keep working out, manage your expectations, and be gentle with yourself. The best part is that *Divine SelfQare* methods can be achieved safely and in a simple way right from the privacy, comfort, and security of your own home, with the help of Queendom Qare. While many of the *Divine SelfQare* strategies and methods can be done in solitude, some of the methods will require assistance. So why not invite a sister-friend to share in the experience of good company and health, as both of you practice *Divine SelfQare* to achieve *Total Body Alignment*?

The Divine SelfQare Strategy proposes a set of wellness protocols to ensure that the organs related to the crown, throne, and pedestal of your temple are in optimal condition. These cleansing routines can be done periodically and whenever you feel the need. Life is hard; at times, we need to give a little extra boost of love, attention, and care to keep the energy flowing in order to fulfill our Divine Purpose as women, daughters, mothers, sisters, and aunts. We must stay alert and ready to meet the needs of our community as healers, businesswomen, inventors, and spiritual sisters to our family, friends, and those near and dear to us.

Divine SelfQare cleanses involve specific tools that you can and should have to support you along your journey. Each of these will be discussed next. Additionally, you should note that any of our effective *Divine SelfQare* treatments usually require a combination of two or more of the four natural elements (**Air, Fire, Earth,** and **Water**). The more elements in your focused cleansing, the greater the outcome, and you will also find it to be a more sensual, rewarding experience. Look for elements in a variety of forms. For instance, *fire* will present as *fire* itself, but it may also be used to create heat, to transform the other elements into steam, or to create a vacuum-like effect when you do our Ear Qleanse treatment. You will interact with the elements in surprising ways as you get familiar with the concept.

More importantly, the act of cleansing is not sufficient in itself. As practitioners of *Divine SelfQare*, we always invite the Most High as the Divine Healer by vocalizing our highest intention. So, with each cleanse, you will find an affirmational prayer to recite before engaging in the physical act of cleansing. Remember, **Divine Intent** is the fifth element. As we discussed in Chapter 5, **Divine Intent** is the mechanism we employ when engaging the art and science of *trans-physics*.

Whether you perform these *Divine SelfQare* strategies on yourself or another person, always recite your intentions in a conversational tone so that they can be heard. This is the key difference between *Divine SelfQare* Practitioners and others. You request the presence of the Most High, who is the ultimate healer, in all activities related to the health and wellness strategies you employ for yourself or on behalf of others.

The reason why the *Divine SelfQare* methods focus more on your head, womb, and feet, is because these become the focal point of keeping your body in its optimal state. We don't think about these areas as much as we should. Hopefully, these *Divine SelfQare Strategies* will be successful in shifting that reality for present and future generations of women.

The diagram below illustrates the relationship between the elements, these bodily focal points, and the outcome we desire - *Total Body Alignment*. As you will see, when the five elements are strategically employed for the care of the crown, throne, and pedestal, what emerges is a woman who experiences *Total Body Alignment*.

The Divine SelfQare Strategy

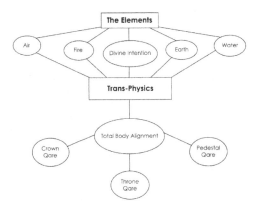

The Sacred Temple

Now, let's briefly review the function of these three focal points of the sacred temple or feminine body.

The Head As A Sacred Crown

Your head is your sacred **Crown**. Therefore, Crown care relates to the process of keeping a healthy head overall, and it mainly consists of managing the functions of sight, hearing, smell & speech. This aspect of the *Divine SelfQare Strategy* focuses on elevation. Just as the outstretched branches of the tree aim to touch the Heavens, the woman's head is as close physically she can be to the Divine. This is why her senses should be at their peak as well. The head or the crown empowers you to think, understand, and provide your body with the strength needed to carry on. Uninterrupted blood flow to the head promotes body and brain health. It allows your nervous system to take control of your body and become more perceptive of the environment around you.

The Womb As A Royal Throne

Every temple has a **Throne**. And your throne relates to the seat of feminine essence and creative reproduction, which generally encompasses the vagina, uterus, and vulva. At Queendom Qare, we often refer to this collection of organs as the *womb*. We mean that in the *trans-physical* sense. Anatomically speaking, the womb refers to the organ that allows for the development of new life. In *trans-physics*, the womb is always active in women who practice *Divine SelfQare*. For us, the *womb* represents the center for all creativity, life, brilliance, and ingenuity; therefore, being in alignment or centered is important for all women to experience *Divine Creativity* and harmony with self, nature, and others.

Just like the crown elevates you when in alignment, the sacred womb is the creative hub and center of your body. It aligns perfectly with your Divine Purpose as a woman.

The Feet As A Grand Pedestal

Pedestal care is all about the feet. Other than the head and the womb, our feet also play an incredibly essential role in our health. Many cultures believe bacteria enter the body through the feet, which explains why paying attention to the health of the feet and keeping them clean and dry is especially important.

Trans-physically speaking, the feet are essential for a sense of grounding and overall life stability. Taking good care of feet increases their strength and flexibility. This, in turn, gives you longer standing hours while you work and take on challenging projects. As women, many of us have responsibilities that require us to stand all day. Be it parenting or conducting meetings, strong, healthy feet are essential.

Divine SelfQare Routine | Schedule

Below you will find the respective cleanses that form the *Divine SelfQare* methods. One can employ these methods at intervals of time for routine wellness, but they can also be employed as deemed necessary to address stressful points in life. The recommended schedule is listed in the diagram below:

CROWN CARE	MINIMALLY	RECOMMENDED
Eye Cleanse	At least 1 time per month	Same
Oral Cleanse	Once every 2 weeks	4 times per month
Ear Cleanse	Once every 3 months	Same
THRONE CARE		
Vaginal Steaming	Twice per month	3 times per month
Jeweling	Twice per month	4-6 times per month
PEDESTAL CARE		
Foot Soak	At least 1 time per month	Same

The schedule above is recommended for usual circumstances or routine care under good health conditions. This may be modified as deemed necessary. Listen to your body and observe good health and hygiene practices. None of the information contained in this guide is meant to serve as a diagnosis, treatment, or cure for any disease or replace standard medical practice that you may have received from your doctor.

Under any circumstances involving poor health or specific medical conditions or complications from the disease, seek the advice of competent medical professionals.

Divine SelfQare Methods

Cleanse The Crown | Achieve Elevation

Eye Qleanse

Not only are the eyes necessary to experience life visually, but they are also important *trans-physically* to interpret the meaning of life and grasp the world's beauty through Divine Vision. Everyday stressors such as pollution present in the environment, digital eye strain, sleep deprivation, and unhealthy diets can have adverse effects on your vision. This impacts your spiritual eyesight in negative ways as well. You may also find that redness, soreness, swelling, puffiness, dryness, or other forms of irritation in or around your eyes can lead to headaches that prevent you from functioning at your best.

The solution for these and many other visual problems is the *Divine SelfQare* strategy referred to as the Thermal Eye Qleanse. It involves using a natural heat source from an organic vegetable heated to a certain temperature before placing it over your clean, closed eyes for twenty minutes. This natural heat-induced eye treatment assists in killing bacteria, fungi, parasites, and viruses that live on or around the eyes.

The Five Elements Involved:

While preparing for the treatment, be mindful of elements involved in the Thermal Eye Qleanse, which are:

- **Air** (Steam will be produced as heat from the potato moves through the eye masks to the eyes.)
- **Fire** (Heat, the primary cleansing agent, is produced by warming a potato in the oven at 350 degrees for 20 minutes.)
- **Earth** (In the form of a potato, represents the vibration of the earth. It will act as a conductor of heat.)

- **Water** (The fusion of the ***air, fire,*** and ***earth*** will increase the presence of the ***water*** element. This will naturally hydrate the eyes while helping to kill bacterial infections and viruses.)
- **Divine Intent** through prayer

How Does It Help

- A *Thermal Eye Treatment* is soothing, detoxifying, and antimicrobial. It helps bring the natural microbes present in and around the eyes into balance and make your eyes feel better right away.
- It can also induce hydration and ease the dryness that sometimes accompanies eye infections.
- It also helps reduce the clogging that occurs from the accumulation of natural oils produced in the glands of the eyelids by thinning the oil, allowing it to drain safely.
- The overall benefits of this amazing, simple earth-based *Thermal Eye Treatment* are plentiful, as people have reported relief from muscle spasms, pain, discomfort from pink eye, and other infections.
- You will feel relaxed and relieved after this eye qleanse treatment.

What Tools You'll Need

- The Queendom Qare Qustom Eye Masq and Eye Qover
- A fresh, organic potato cut in half
- A heat source (oven is best - microwaving is acceptable only when necessary)
- A few drops of coconut oil

How To Conduct A Thermal Eye Qleanse

1. Wash the potato and cut it in half.

2. Place the two halves of the potato on a clean baking sheet lined with parchment paper and bake at 350 degrees for 20 minutes.

3. Remove the potato halves from the oven and carefully wrap each one separately in a paper towel until completely covered; then place them on a plate and set aside until ready to use.

4. Position your supplies next to your bed or massage table.

5. Place the potatoes neatly inside of the inserts located on the backside of the Queendom Qare EyeMasq.

6. Place the Queendom Qare Eye Qover over your eyes to serve as a barrier that helps to protect your skin and evenly distribute the heat. (You can test the temperature of the heated potatoes on your wrist prior to placing it on your eyes.)

7. Next, carefully place the Eye Masq with the heated potato halves inserted directly over the Eye Qover, pull the elastic band over your head to secure the Eye Masq in place. The elastic band of the Eye Masq should be positioned above your ears.

8. Align the circumference of the potato halves directly over the eyes, flat side down. If too hot, remove the Masq and let it cool down for 2-3 minutes.

9. Once at a comfortable temperature, lie down again, apply the Eye Masq and Qover, and enjoy a thermal eye treatment uninterrupted for 20 minutes.

10. Remove the Eye Masq and protective Eye Qover, apply a drop of coconut oil to the eyelids, massage the oil gently with your index finger, and relax for an additional 10 minutes.

Affirmation/Prayer

"I cleanse my eyes to remove impurities so that I may come before you, Most High, with a clean heart and pure spirit. Perfect my eyesight and bless me with Divine Vision so that I may see the path that leads to the fulfillment of my Divine Purpose."

Estimated Time To Complete

1 hour

Ear Qleanse

The ear is not only a source of hearing, but it is also responsible for maintaining a sense of balance in your body. The ear canal can often get blocked with impurities such as wax, yeast, debris, and micro-parasites that can travel from the sinuses, which must be removed for clear hearing, balanced movement, and comfort.

Candling or *Qandling* is a non-invasive procedure that has been long in use by the indigenous people of ancient Africa, Asia, and early Americans for hygiene and spiritual healing. The process can take up to 40 minutes, and it involves using a burning candle surrounded by a protective disc and placing it into the ear canal vertically while you lie on your side. The benefits of this treatment include relief from sinus infections, itchy ears, and headaches while also having a restorative effect on your sense of balance.

The Five Elements Involved:

While preparing for the treatment, be mindful of the elements involved in an Ear Qleanse which are:

- **Air** (in the form of Smoke)
- **Fire** (in its own form used to light the Ear Qone/ Qandle)
- **Earth** (Natural Qones/ Qandles crafted from Beeswax)

- **Water** (in its natural form to extinguish the *fire*)
- **Divine Intent** through prayer

How Does It Help

Ear Candling/Qandling or Coning/Qoning can relieve pain and irritation resulting from:

- Sinus congestion
- Colds
- Earaches and infections
- Candida
- Excess wax buildup

What You'll Need

1. Queendom Qare Ear Qones/Qandles
2. Ear Oil (optional)
3. Heat resistant cloth or small towel
4. A cup of water to extinguish the fire
5. Scissors
6. A lighter
7. Heat resistant Candle plate
8. A second person must conduct this cleanse (preferably another *Divine SelfQare Practitioner*)

How To Conduct An Ear Qleanse

1. Lay on your side as you rest on a massage table with your head on a pillow.
2. Place the tapered end of the hollowed qone made from cotton and beeswax gently inside the ear.
3. Light the other end to produce the heat from the top of the qandle to create a vacuum-pulling effect.
4. For safety purposes, use a candle plate to deflect heat from the flame and collect candle debris.

5. When the Qandle burns down to no less than two inches, remove the Qandle, extinguish the flame in the glass of water, place a piece of cotton over the ear canal to collect any residue that proceeds from the ear and repeat the process on the other side.
6. Note: Expect to hear a crackling, suction sound during the treatment; it is normal and relaxing.

Affirmational Prayer

"I cleanse my ears to remove impurities so that I may come before you, Most High, with a clean heart and pure spirit. Perfect my hearing and give me Divine Listening gifts so that I may hear the sound of your first voice as I fulfill my Divine Purpose."

Estimated Time To Complete

35-40 minutes

Oral Qleanse

The mouth is responsible for speech or verbal expression, which is one of our main forms of communication. The mouth can become a source of bacteria and other microbes that can negatively impact your oral health and disrupt your internal balance.

Oil pulling is used to remove impurities or detox your mouth by removing the layer of biofilm with a special blend of natural and therapeutic oils that can refresh and reinvigorate your mouth cavity. *Divine SelfQare* practitioners should have good oral health for overall well-being.

The Three Elements Involved:

While preparing for the treatment, be mindful of the elements involved in an Oral Qleanse, which are:

- **Earth** (the oil from a coconut represents the element of earth, bringing healing agents and antimicrobials that remove bacteria and lauric acid that strengthens the teeth)
- **Water** (the water itself used to rinse any oil residue that remains after completion of the pull)
- **Divine Intent** through prayer

How Does It Help

Oil pulling can relieve oral discomfort and pain resulting from:

- Harmful bacteria in your mouth
- Bad breath
- Inflammation and infections
- What You'll Need
- Oral Qleanse Pulling Oils By Queendom Qare (*Forever Floral, Mint Maker,* or *Super Spice*)
- Water to rinse after brushing

How To Conduct An Oral Qleanse

- Measure 1-2 Tablespoons of Oral Qleanse Pulling Oil By Queendom Qare
- Swish vigorously around the mouth for at least 20 minutes
- Spit the solution out into a disposal container (not the sink or toilet)
- Rinse your mouth thoroughly with warm water
- Brush your teeth gently, then rinse again with warm water

Affirmational Prayer

"I cleanse my mouth to remove impurities so that I may come before you, Most High, with a clean heart and pure spirit. Perfect my words and bless

me with Divine Oratory so that I may speak sacred life over your people as I fulfill my Divine Purpose."

Estimated Time To Complete

20 - 25 minutes

Nasal & Upper Respiratory Qleanse | Facial Detox

The face and nose play a key role in beauty and health. Having a facial can not only improve the appearance and feel of the skin on the face and neck by detoxing the pores, but it can also clear out and kill bacteria or viruses that attach themselves to the soft tissue in the nose and throat with heat, herbs, and steam. Purified skin and nasal passages can make you feel lighter, better, and also promote better sleep. Not only does your skin glow, but the reduced sebum protection also keeps acne and blackheads at bay.

The Qrown Qare system of wellness affords women to enjoy a powerful and relaxing facial steam or upper respiratory qleanse from the safety and comfort of home. The Crown or Qrown as we like to say at Queendom Qare, is the elevating function of the head for *Total Body Alignment*. When a woman's head, including her eyes, ears, nose, and mouth, can function properly, she can see, hear, smell, breath, taste, speak and even face the world in a confident effort to achieve her goals and fulfill her *Divine Purpose.*

The Five Elements Involved:

While preparing for the treatment, be mindful of the elements involved in a Facial Detox | Upper Respiratory | Nasal Qleanse, which are:

- **Air** (in the form of Steam)
- **Fire** (in its own form used to boil the water)
- **Earth** (essential oils and/or herbal blends)
- **Water** (in its own form)
- **Divine Intent** through prayer

How Does It Help

Facial Steaming and Upper Respiratory | Nasal Qleanses can provide multiple benefits Including:

- Purifies the skin on the face
- Opens and detoxifies pores
- Fights colds and flu virus
- Cleanses the nostrils
- Combats upper respiratory infections

What You'll Need

1. Crown/Qrown Qare Steam Station (patent pending)
2. Therapeutic Grade Essential Oils (peppermint, eucalyptus, thieves blend) and/or a Qrown Qare Herbal Blend
3. Small pot or bowl
4. Hot Water

How To Conduct A Facial Steam | Nasal Qleanse

1. Place the Crown/Qrown Qare Steam Station on a countertop or table.
2. Bring a small pot of water to a boil. You only need a few cups of water.
3. Wash your face with a gentle cleanser while the water is heating to remove makeup and dirt.
4. Once the water reaches a boil, add a few drops of essential oil and/or a Crown/Qrown Qare Herbal Blend.
5. Put the pot of water into the Crown/Qrown Qare Steam Station directly over the heat-resistant cork barrier.
6. Close the lid and place the cotton Plush Facial Pillow on top of the Crown/Qrown Qare Steam Station lid.
7. Check the temperature for comfort by holding your face or hand over the pillow at a safe distance. Allow to cool if necessary, before steaming.

8. Sit or stand in front of the Crown/Qrown Qare Steam Station to engage in steaming by placing your face over the pillow and relaxing over the warm steam for 15-20 minutes.

Affirmational Prayer

"I cleanse my face, nose, and upper respiratory system so that I may come before you, Most High, with a clean heart and pure spirit. Perfect my breathing and detoxify my pores so that I may face the world with your blessings and inhale the scent of the kingdom of light in my nostrils as I work to fulfill my Divine Purpose."

Estimated Time To Complete

35-40 minutes total

Cleanse The Throne | Achieve Centering

Welcome Womb Wellness

This method of centering women in themselves through steaming is based on the ancient wisdom of working with the four elements – **air, fire, earth,** and **water**. This ancient science can help you unlock your creative potential and access the source of your feminine essence. Even though modern medicine has just begun to acknowledge the practice, African women from Mozambique to Ghana, from Nigeria to Ethiopia, and other regions of the continent have been tapping into the secret health benefits of vaginal steaming or smoking for millennia.

The wellness practice allows for feminine healing and vaginal resilience by cleansing and restoring the uterus and vaginal walls. By exposing these sacred areas to gentle herbal steam, women are able to center themselves in divine creativity and restore their sense of wellness from within.

There are many ways in which we as women can feel out of alignment. Throne or womb imbalance is one of the biggest reasons. What else can cause us to feel vaginal pain and discomfort? At least five common types of vaginal trauma or injuries are likely to impact every woman at some point in her life. Trauma has multiple meanings, but in this context, vaginal *"trauma"* refers to the medical aspect of the word *"trauma,"* which means a serious injury to a person's body. This is NOT a discussion about the kind of trauma that leads to emotional harm. There is a place for that conversation later on, but not for this type of therapeutic discussion.

Here is what you should know about five common types of vaginal trauma or injury:

The Top 5 Challenges to Being Centered In Vaginal Wellness

1. *The First Type of Vaginal Trauma Relates To Situations Arising From Sexual intercourse*

   This can happen to women during passionate sex when friction from penetration can create tears inside the vagina. This is likely to happen if the sensitive tissues that form the vaginal wall have not been sufficiently lubricated. Sometimes vaginal trauma can happen when the penis comes into direct contact with the cervix. If the woman is not in a state of arousal, this contact may result in a bruised cervix.

2. *The Second Type of Vaginal Trauma Stems From Injuries That Occur During Childbirth*

   Vaginal trauma can sometimes occur due to the stretching of the pelvic floor during delivery. Since the pelvic floor is responsible for urination control and holds the pelvic organs in place, women can experience specific problems if the pelvic floor is weakened by the stress associated with stretching during childbirth and delivery. These can sometimes include distortion of the vagina; vaginal heaviness, or a sensation of dragging, pain associated with sexual intercourse; urine, gas, or stool incontinence; or scarring of the vaginal tissue if it required stitches.

3. *The Third Type of Trauma Stems From A Type of Surgery Known As A Vaginal Hysterectomy*

Hysterectomies are a common surgery. Over 20 million women in the US have had one, and about 12% of these took place between 2006 and 2010 on women between the ages of 40 and 44. Although a vaginal hysterectomy is shown to be the most cost-effective of the five forms of surgical hysterectomies, it comes with a serious risk of shortening or damaging the vagina.

4. *The Fourth Class of Vaginal Trauma You Should Be Aware Is Likely To Occur From The Loss of Virginity*

Technically, virgins are females who meet certain physical characteristics - namely an intact hymen. There are more than eight types of hymen, which is a thin fold of mucous membrane (about 1mm thick) covering the vagina. A virgin is likely to experience pain the first time she has sexual intercourse as the hymen tissue and other vaginal organs expand during this first sexual encounter.

5. The Final Type of Vaginal Trauma Happens During and After An Abortion

Women who undergo medical or surgical abortion, regardless of the reason and irrespective of their political perspective or moral code, have experienced tremendous vaginal or womb trauma. In fact, heavy bleeding for up to 2 weeks after the completion of surgical or medical abortion is considered normal. Abortion interrupts the natural reproductive cycle, which will have huge physical, emotional, and mental consequences.

Womb Qleanse Vaginal Steaming As An At-Home Therapeutic Treatment

Vaginal steaming can have powerful and reinvigorating effects on your cervix as the steam can carry the essence of the herbs to spread its benefits. There is a proper process that must be followed to get the most out of this health practice, which incorporates the elements of **Air, Fire, Earth**, and **Water.** I will share the details so you can cleanse and restore the uterus and vagina by exposing them to the gentle, powerful, therapeutic, and healing properties of herbal steam.

The Five Elements Involved:

While preparing for the treatment, be mindful of the elements involved in a Womb/Vaginal Qleanse:

- **Air** (This element is present in the form of steam created by the fusion of heat and moisture to carry healing properties of nature into the woman's vaginal opening and into the pores of the vulva)
- **Fire** (This element is first present as itself when boiling/simmering the water and plants, then it translates through the remaining heat that circulates the warm air to facilitate the cleanse during this hydrotherapy session)
- **Earth** (This element is present in herbs, plants, and spices contained in one of four Queendom Qare offerings for womb wellness: Qleanse, Qondition, Qonquer & Qontrol Herbal blends)
- **Water** (This element is present as itself through the preparation of the hydrotherapy session)
- **Divine Intent** through prayer.

How Does It Help?

Ease the pain and discomfort from

1. The five common types of vaginal trauma
2. Menstrual cycle pain and PMS
3. UTI/Yeast Infections
4. Postpartum Stress
5. Restoring Balance Post Sexual Intercourse

What You'll Need

1. A Throne Qare Steam Station
2. A Queendom Qare Steam Gown
3. A Plush Pillow For Steaming
4. Queendom Qare Herbal Blends To Qleanse, Qondition, Qonquer, or Qontrol
5. A pot of steamy, hot water
6. Fresh Towels
7. A quiet, clean at-home spa or designated area
8. Privacy
9. A cup of tea (can be made from the organic herbal blends used for steaming)

Affirmational Prayer

"I cleanse my womb to remove impurities so that I may come before you, Most High, with a clean heart and pure spirit. Perfect my reproductive gifts and bless me with Divine Creativity so that I may develop the kind of solutions that honor, protect, and perpetuate life and enable me to fulfill my Divine Purpose."

Estimated Time To Complete

1 hour (prep and steam session)

Special Disclaimer | Do Not Steam If Any Of the Following Circumstances Apply To You:
1. Pregnancy
2. Menstruation
3. Recent Insemination has occurred while actively trying to conceive a baby
4. Longer than usual menstrual cycles or multiple cycles within a month.
5. Active STD or STI

The Art of Jeweling

A more proactive form of womb wellness is a therapeutic set of exercises using pure rose quartz as a weight to strengthen the pelvic floor and gain other benefits by healing the womb area and vagina at a deeper level.

Rose quartz is the stone selected for *Divine SelfQare* practitioners for its gentle feel, soft color, cool sensation, and welcoming touch. It is a natural stone that centers the woman's core and helps to calm the nerves after a stressful day. The rose quartz jewel comes in different sizes, challenging the muscles of the pelvic floor. It is recommended that a beginner starts with a larger size and work their way towards a smaller stone, as muscles that form the vaginal wall master retention of the stone under a variety of circumstances like walking, standing, or when completing the Queendom Qare guided pelvic floor exercises.

The Four Elements Involved:

While preparing for the treatment, be mindful of the elements involved in Jeweling:

- **Air** (This element is present in the focused breathing of the woman as she aligns her inhales and exhales in

tune with the squeeze and release of the pelvic floor muscles)
- **Earth** (This element is present in the purity of the crystal which is always certified as pure rose quartz by the Gemological Institute of America)
- **Water** (This element is present as itself through the pure waters stimulated by the exposing the precious Jewel to sunlight after washing, drying and storing properly)
- **Divine Intent** through prayer

How Does It Help

1. **Balance:** Rose quartz is a powerful tool of wellness, and it can be used to re-center yourself to optimal performance through Divine restoration.
2. **Strength:** Jeweling is an effective way to increase the strength of your vaginal muscles through pelvic exercises that engage your inner core and enhance physical and emotional well-being.
3. **Well-being:** Jeweling helps you create a routine that focuses you in prioritizing your overall health and wellness.
4. **Creativity:** The womb is a sacred space that is important to the creative process as it holds, secures, nurtures, and gives birth to both ideas and life. Jeweling supports and strengthens reproductive health
5. **Sensuality:** By jeweling, you can mindfully and routinely enhance and develop an awareness of your feminine essence to feel more attractive, healthy, precious, and experience greater Divine Intimacy.

What You'll Need

1. A Queendom Qare Throne Jewel (GIA certified Rose Quartz)
2. Water

3. Natural liquid soap
4. Warm water
5. Therapeutic grade lemon essential oil or Himalayan sea salt
6. Natural cotton cloth (optional)
7. A safe stable storage case

How To Prep & Insert Your Throne Jewel

1. Cleanse
   - **Throne Jewels** need a thorough cleansing before use.
   - First, wash your precious Jewel with a natural liquid soap under warm, running water.
   - Next, place the Jewel in a bowl of warm sea salt water for a minimum of 5 hours.
   - Rinse thoroughly and allow the air to dry (preferably in an area where it can be exposed to sunlight).

2. Bless
   - After cleaning, you should bless your Jewel.
   - This should be done prior to each use.
   - Simply petition the blessings of the Most High over your effort to secure the health and vitality of the womb using your Jewel as an aide to strengthen and support your pelvic floor with jeweling exercises.

3. Insert and Use
   - Inserting a Jewel, whether drilled/strung or undrilled, is similar to putting a tampon in.
   - If the Jewel is drilled, first thread the hemp strand into the hole and make sure the length permits you to draw the Jewel out after the exercise is finished.
   - Then, carefully and gently direct the Jewel into your vagina with the drilled (or smaller) side down.

- When inserting the Jewel, it's important to remember that the bigger component goes in first.
- Then perform the Jeweling exercise of your choice.
- Don't worry about losing your Jewel; the cervix works as a barrier to keep the Jewel in the vaginal canal during the activity.

How To Exercise The Jewel

Now that your Jewel is in place, make good use of it with some pelvic floor strengthening exercises. Be sure to select a private and comfortable spot on the floor or any other level surface, such as a patch of grass. Take your time to get comfortable with the exercises and try to ensure you get at least 15 minutes of peace and quiet, so you can begin your journey towards health and healing.

Exercise 1

1. **Position 1a)** To start this exercise, lie on your back, and bend your knees with your feet flat on the floor.
2. Take three deep breaths.

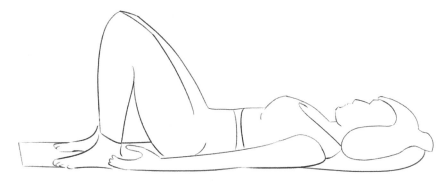

3. **Position 1b)** On the third exhale, position your hands behind your knees, gently bring your knees together, and lift your feet off the floor until you form about a 60-degree angle with your knees.

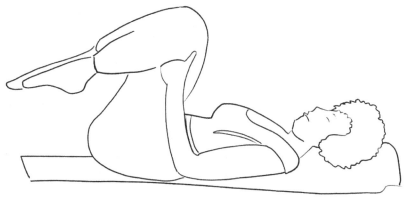

4. Now that you are settled into this position squeeze and hold the Jewel with your vagina for 5 seconds.

5. Then relax for 5 seconds before going back to **Position 1a)** by slowly lowering your feet back to the ground when done.

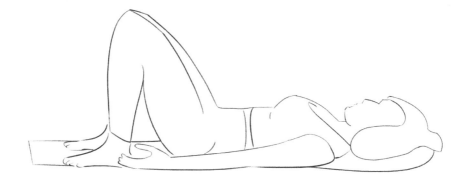

6. Repeat this exercise routine 10 times.
7. Gradually increase the number of seconds that you squeeze the Jewel until you reach 10 seconds by the end of the routine.

Exercise 2

1. **Position 2a)** To start this exercise, lie on your back, bend your knees, position your heels as close to your buttocks as possible, and place your feet flat on the floor.

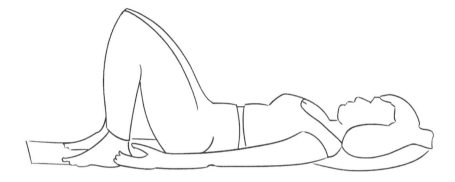

2. Take three deep breaths.
3. **Position 2b)** On the third exhale, press your feet and arms into the floor and push your tailbone towards the sky as you lift your buttocks off the floor.

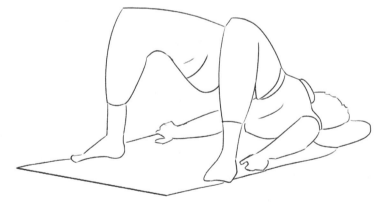

4. Keep your thighs and feet parallel.
5. Squeeze the Jewel with your vagina, hold each squeeze for 5 seconds, and then relax for 5 seconds.
6. Do this squeeze and release 10 times.

7. Back to **Position 2a)** When done, slowly lower your buttocks back to the floor, and relax your spine.

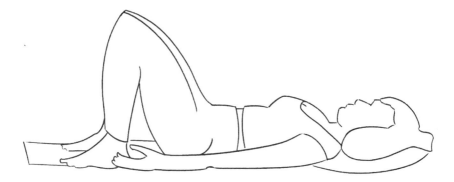

8. Repeat this entire exercise routine 4 more times.

Exercise 3

1. **Position 3a)** To start this exercise, lie on your back, spread your legs and feet apart.

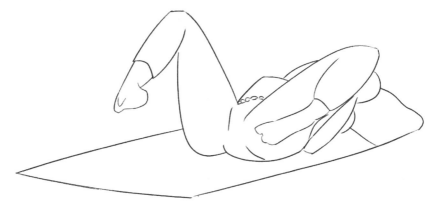

2. Bend your knees toward your chest so that your toes point opposite the crown of your head and your knees align with your shoulders.
3. Slowly take three deep breaths.
4. **Position 3b)** On the third inhale, lift your feet up and out toward your head so that your legs form a wide "V" shape.

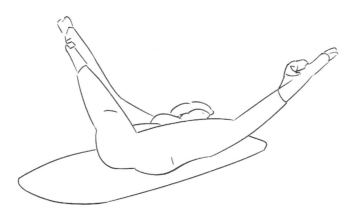

5. Then grab the heels of your feet and hold the position.

6. As you settle into the position, squeeze, and release the Jewel with your vagina.
7. Repeat this sequence 10 times.
8. Back to **Position 3a)** When done, slowly release your feet from your hands and lower your feet back to the floor.

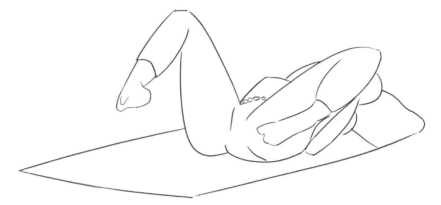

9. Repeat this entire routine up to 10 times.

Exercise 4

1. **Position 4a)** Start on your hands and knees in a "tabletop" position.

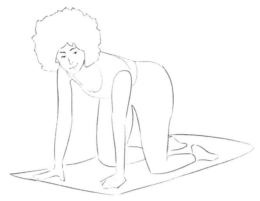

2. Make sure your knees are set directly below your hips and that your wrists, elbows, and shoulders are in line and perpendicular to the floor.
3. Center your head in a neutral position, eyes looking at the floor.
4. Take three deep breaths.
5. On the third inhale, move into **Position 4b)** so that you lift your buttocks and chest toward the ceiling, allowing your belly to sink toward the floor.

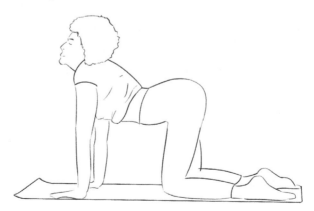

6. Lift your head to look straight ahead. As you settle into this position, squeeze, and release the Jewel 3 times.
7. Inhaling as you squeeze, exhaling as you release.
8. Back to **Position 4a)** Breathe and exhale as you return to the neutral "tabletop" position on your hands and knees.

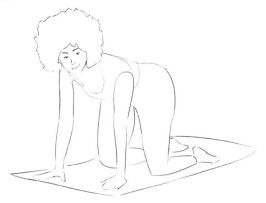

9. Repeat the entire routine 10 times.

Exercise 5

1. **Position 5a)** Start on your hands and knees in a "tabletop" position.

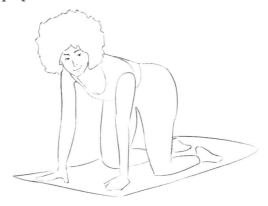

2. Make sure your knees are set directly below your hips and that your wrists, elbows, and shoulders are in line and perpendicular to the floor.
3. Center your head in a neutral position, eyes looking at the floor.
4. Take three deep breaths.
5. On the third exhale, move into **Position 5b)** so that you round your spine toward the ceiling, making sure to keep your shoulders and knees in position.

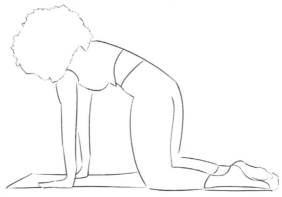

6. Release your head toward the floor, but do not force your chin to your chest.

7. As you settle into this position, squeeze, and release the Jewel 3 times.
8. Inhale as you squeeze, exhale as you release.
9. Back to **Position 5a)** On the next inhale, return to the neutral "tabletop" position on your hands and knees.

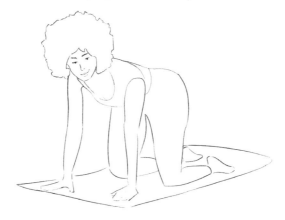

10. Repeat the entire routine 10 times.
11. Note: As you advance in jeweling, another technique is to go directly from position 4b to 5b by inhaling on 4 and exhaling on 5. Repeat 10 times.

How To Remove & Cleanse Your Throne Jewel

After a refreshing exercise session, don't forget to remove and clean your Jewel thoroughly so it can be ready to use before your next session.

1. Remove
   - Removing your Throne Jewel is simple.
   - Relax and take a few deep breaths.
   - Get into a squatted position and push out with your vaginal muscles.
   - If needed, you may use your fingers to scoop the Jewel out or gently pull the string so that it glides out slowly if you use one.
   - You can also do a little jump up and down to help move the Jewel down the vaginal canal before removing it.

2. Disinfect And Store
   - Remove the string (if drilled) and wash the Jewel with gentle natural soap under warm running water.
   - To disinfect, place the clean Jewel into a bowl of warm water containing two drops of therapeutic grade lemon essential oil or a teaspoon of Himalayan sea salt for up to 5 hours.
   - Allow to dry in the sunlight (if possible), or simply pat dry with a lint-free natural cotton cloth.
   - Store your Jewel away from other items that can cause cracks or breakage.

Affirmational Prayer

"I use this Throne Jewel to strengthen my sacred womb through strategic pelvic floor exercises so that with your blessings, Oh Most High, I will experience youthful vitality and Divine Creativity

to aid me in the fulfillment of my Divine Purpose as a result of all my many wellness efforts."

Estimated Time To Complete

15 - 30 minutes (may use longer, visit queendomqare.com for more information.)

Cleanse The Pedestal | Achieve Grounding

Focus On Feet

As women, we may feel compelled to expose ourselves to salon treatments to get pedicures, manicures, and worse, artificial nail sets. These practices can be dangerous hygienically due to the fact that these establishments use toxic materials to achieve these ends. But how can you care for your feet if you're exposing them to dangerous chemicals?

The environment of these salons is also not conducive to healing foot treatments as commercial foot care is eventually detrimental to your health. Even if we think our skin feels good at that moment, trust me when I tell you, time will show the damage that these treatments have on our feet. For this reason, it is more suitable for us to focus on more natural treatments that focus on incorporating the four elements of **Air, Fire, Earth** and **Water.**

Foot Qleanse

A *pedestal or foot qleanse* can provide some much-needed relief from staying on your feet all day. The benefits of a foot soak are enhanced by the introduction of herbal blends and salts to soothe and soften the feet. Even a 20-minute soak can release any tension you're carrying around in your feet, and you can complete the process by applying oils to lock in the benefits. Once the treatment is completed, you can stand firmly and remain grounded in pursuit of fulfilling your Divine Purpose.

The Four Elements Involved:

While preparing for the treatment, be mindful of the elements involved in this *Pedestal Qleanse*, which are:

- **Fire** (This element is present as itself when boiling/simmering the water and ginger root and/herbal blends)
- **Earth** (This element is present in the organic salts, plants, spices, herbs, and essential oil)
- **Water** (This element is present at itself to facilitate the cleanse)
- **Divine Intent** through prayer

How Does It Help

- Tired, aching, swollen feet
- Stress and muscle tension
- Sense of instability

What You'll Need

- A foot basin or large bowl
- *Queendom Qare Foot Soak Blend*
- Therapeutic-grade Ginger essential oil (*Young Living* preferred) and/or a large piece of fresh ginger root
- Coconut oil for moisturizer
- 2-3 Clean Towels

How To Conduct A Pedestal Soak

- In a large pot, add a large piece of fresh ginger, 1 cup of the Queendom Qare Herbal Ginger-Mint Foot and Ankle Blend and fill with water. Bring to a boil, and then simmer for 15 minutes. Turn off the stove and allow cooling down for 10 to 20 minutes.

- Fold a large, thick towel in half and place it on the floor in front of your chair
- Place an empty Queendom Qare foot basin over the towel and slowly fill with heated ginger, herbal water no more than 100 degrees Fahrenheit (use a thermometer if one is available or test the temperature of the water by placing a drop or two on your wrist)
- Add 1 cup of the Foot Soak Salts & Herbs by Queendom Qare
- Stir and allow to dissolve
- Put your feet into the basin
- Cover your feet and the basin with another towel to trap in the heat but try to keep the towel dry
- Soak for 20 minutes
- Dry your feet completely paying attention to the spaces between the toes
- Gently massage your feet with 5 drops of Ginger oil per foot then moisturize with a few drops of organic coconut oil

Affirmational Prayer

"I cleanse my feet to remove impurities so that I may come before you, Most High, with a clean heart and pure spirit. Set my feet in the right direction and bless me to feel grounded. Heavenly One, please guide me along the path that leads to my Divine Purpose."

Estimated Time To Complete

1 hour

The Tools Of Wellness Through Divine SelfQare

Every woman deserves to experience Divine Health. It is her Divine Birthright, but in this modern world, we as women still have to fight for it...we have to fight for our birthright!

We are at a point where I have to ensure that I provide all my readers with a path to follow – a path that will lead them to Divine Health through adopting *The Divine SelfQare Strategy*.

Here, I want to take out some time to talk about the power of Divine Health which is a gift from the Most High to our minds, spirits, and bodies. Divine Health is defined as being in excellent physical condition, possessing a sound mind, and experiencing spiritual balance at any age.

In this manner, the tools, and products that I am going to speak to you about help us achieve everything that is sacred to a practitioner of *Divine SelfQare*.

Queendom Qare focuses on the preservation of health through natural healing modalities. This online store can help women retrieve the specific tools of natural healing and wellness that help to facilitate *Divine SelfQare* methods outlined in this book.

As a *Divine SelfQare Strategist*, and the creator of *The Divine SelfQare Strategy*, I am pleased to share my gifts with you, Daughters of the Most High, as you set out to establish a tranquil at-home spa in your own home.

The following items discussed in the methods above will be the best tools you can use in carrying out the *Divine SelfQare Strategy*. Using these tools for all your natural wellness methods will give you the control you need over your own health. You will have your personal armada through which you can safely enjoy the methods of the *Divine SelfQare Strategy*, as we have discussed.

The product lines at Queendom Qare are divided according to the body parts they serve. Here you will find everything you will need for sacred wellness practices regarding the crown, throne, and pedestal.

It's time to adorn your temple with everything Queendom Qare has to offer!

Qrown Qare

An essential product line for a healthy head

Eye Masq

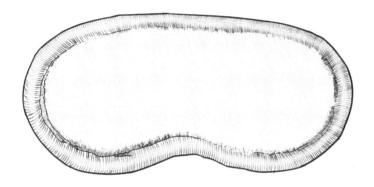

The Eye Masq is a perfect tool for *Divine SelfQare* practitioners seeking to engage in our Thermal Eye Qleanse for optimal health goals. The Purity Masq is designed to enable clean eye health by facilitating thermal eye treatments when used in conjunction with the basic Eye Qover. The special Queendom Qare design of this Eye Masq is perfect for our special earth-based heat qleanse system, giving your eyes the most delicate and special care they deserve.

Oral Qare Cleansers

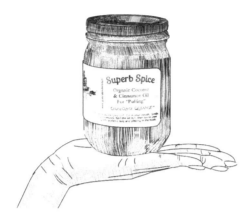

Queendom Qare offers natural Oral Qare Cleansers so that you can try the ancient practice of oil pulling to remove the bacterial biofilm, improve dental health, promote oral hygiene, and eliminate bad breath. Queendom Qare uses an exclusive blend of coconut and essential oils to offer a relaxing and refreshing oral rinse.

What makes the Oral Qleansers most suitable for your Divine Health is that they are free of alcohol, artificial colors, and added flavors. The all-natural blend uses organic coconut oil and an assortment of therapeutic essential oils to achieve the desired taste and mouth feel.

These safe and natural oil pulling rinses are available in several flavors, such as Mint Maker and Superb Spice.

Mint Maker is the perfect way to refresh your oral hygiene and revitalize your taste buds. Whether it's before a meal or a speaking engagement, this can most definitely serve as a confidence booster, making your breath smell fresh all day!

Superb Spice, on the other hand, is excellent for combating bacterial infections, speeding the healing of open sores inside the mouth, and destroying germs that cause bad breath.

Ear Qones or Ear Qandles

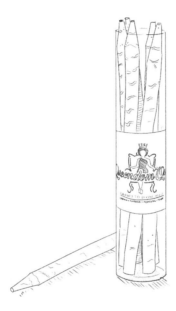

Ear Qones or Ear Qandles are a perfect way to clear build-up in the ear canal and draw out impurities from within. Moreover, they provide a balancing, calming, and therapeutic experience for everyone who wants to enjoy natural wellness methods. You too can enjoy a relaxing candling experience with Queendom Qare premium-quality candles.

Made with food-grade paraffin, beeswax, organic cotton, and a therapeutic combination of 100% pure tea tree, lavender, eucalyptus, or peppermint essential oils, Queendom Qare Ear Qones or Qandles are perfect for those who prioritize clarity and Divine Listening.

Qrown Qare Steam Station

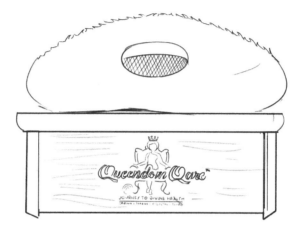

The Crown/Qrown Qare Steam Station (Patent Application No. 63/285,198) is handcrafted for the specific purpose of conducting a steam cleans for the face as well as the nasal passages. It enables *Divine SelfQare* practitioners to safely inhale steam from a bowl of hot water infused with herbs and/or essential oils to facilitate plant-based herbal remedies designed to fight off viruses and bacterial infections that cause upper respiratory disease. It can be used to combat the flu, colds, COVID-19 and similar conditions that may soon arise.

The Queendom Qare Qrown Qare Steam Station is lightweight and constructed with side handles for easy accessibility. The size is perfect for counters and tabletops, making it a great resource for small, compact spaces or larger at home spa areas. Your Crown/Qrown Qare Steam Station Kit comes with a lid and a plush pillow.

The Divine SelfQare Strategy recommends that every Queendom Qare At-Home Spa include a Crown/Qrown Qare Steam Station as an essential part of head or crown wellness. It is necessary for your *Divine SelfQare* routines – especially when it comes to crown/qrown elevation, skin care, and upper respiratory detoxification. Plus, it is a powerful relaxation aide as well.

Throne Qare

Superior quality products for womb wellness

Throne Qare Steam Station

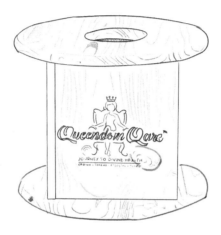

With the help of a Throne Qare Steam Station, women can engage in the sacred form of hydrotherapy known as vaginal steaming in the comfort of their homes.

Through this portable and effective design, it is now possible for you to engage in *Divine SelfQare* whenever you need to rebalance and rejuvenate your womb while you replenish feminine sensuality.

With the help of the Queendom Qare Steam Station, you get to enhance your health, cleanse, condition and control your sacred vaginal parts, while honoring your womb and feminine needs anytime you want.

Plush Pillow

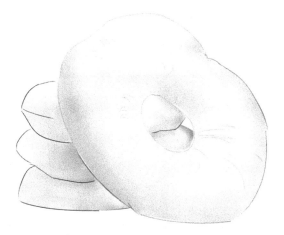

The Throne Qare Steam Plush Pillow is a luxurious pillow to make sure you enjoy every second of your at-home steaming session. The pillow truly enhances the intimacy of your *SelfQare* moment and perfectly seals in the heat while maximizing your comfort. It's lightweight, washable, spa-quality, and stunningly beautiful.

At Queendom Qare, we are all about powerful natural wellness that goes hand in hand with your comfort, which is why this one-size-fits-all plush pillow is made with 100% cotton that is responsibly and safely sourced from the very best.

Herbal Blends

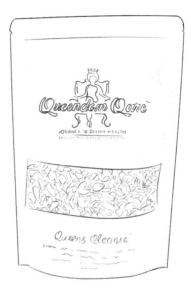

The Throne Qare Steam Station is incomplete without the Throne Qare Herbal Blends. Reap the benefits of the therapeutic smoky essence of Queendom Qare Herbal Blends as they travel with the steam and enter your body to produce wellness.

Not only do you benefit from the medicinal healing of our potent herbal blends, but it also aids immense relaxation. The balanced combination of herbs produces a gentle cleansing effect for overall womb and vaginal wellness, making it an essential product to start your *Divine SelfQare* journey.

Throne Jewels

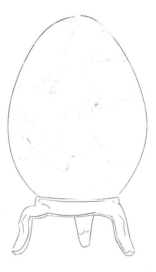

Queendom Qare Throne Jewels are certified by *The Gemological Institute of America* to provide you with only the best Rose Quartz. Throne Jewels offer various therapeutic benefits to Daughters of the Most High who use them responsibly.

They can help tone and strengthen your pelvic floor muscles and promote better reproductive health. Throne Jewels enhance your womb wellness and can help ease pelvic tension. Queendom Qare unique Throne Jewel exercises offer a way to experience a reduction in incontinence, strengthen and rejuvenate pelvic muscles, and heighten your sensual awareness.

Steam Gown

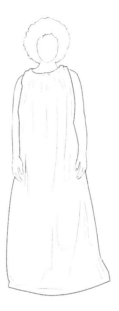

Every woman needs a gorgeous, flowing gown to wear while she revives the essence of her femininity. When seated on your Throne Qare Steam Station, feeling comfortable, safe, and warm is of the utmost importance, which is why the Steam Gown is an essential aspect of the womb hydrotherapy experience. It captures the heat and, in most cases, covers the entire Throne Qare Steam Station!

The Queendom Qare Steam Gown is handmade with gorgeous, soft, and pure white cotton fabric for gentle vaginal steaming or meditative healing. Your Throne will feel the warmth as your gown captures the steam, all while caressing your skin in a blanket of blissful comfort.

Pedestal Qare

Only the best for healthy supple feet

Foot Basin

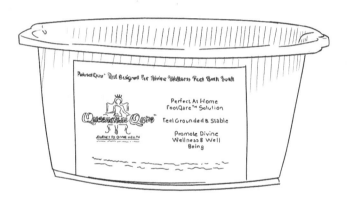

Just like the Throne Qare Steam Station, the Queendom Qare Foot Basin is another product designed to keep your convenience and comfort in mind. The large foot pool is constructed to make your feet feel like they are traveling far away from stress, weight, and pain. Best of all, it's leak-free, portable, and light-weight for you to easily use anywhere around the house.

Foot Soak Salts

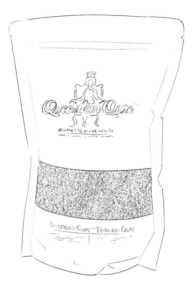

The Queendom Qare Foot Soak is a blend of tantalizing salts and earthy herbs for the therapeutic benefits that your feet crave. When used with warm water, the Foot Soak allows you to relax and unwind as you soothe dry, tired feet. Not only does it rejuvenate your feet, but it also makes them feel strong and stable enough to give you a firm footing.

Immerse Yourself In Wellness

Divine SelfQare Practitioners seek to fulfill their Divine Purpose in life, knowing that being in complete harmony with themselves through *Total Body Alignment* is the way. By focusing on improving the health of your physical body, you can elevate your spiritual and emotional self. Queendom Qare paves the way for you to use the *Divine SelfQare Strategy* as a way to reclaim, restore, replenish, and rejuvenate yourself as you embark on a lifelong wellness journey of the body, mind, and spirit.

The methods you have read about in this book, have been thoughtfully devised and require a set of tools to employ in the execution of the *Divine SelfQare Strategy*. These methods are designed to achieve *Total Body Alignment* or to elevate, center, and ground your head, womb, and feet, respectively.

The unique tools described herein are the best way to facilitate our *Divine SelfQare* strategies and methods and create harmony within. There is no substitute for using them. Collectively, these tools make up the Queendom Qare assets or the custom line of products specifically handcrafted with the highest quality measures that range from sourcing to structural design.

Whether using pure essential oils, natural cotton, organic herbs, or pure pinewood, each of our special assets or products is handcrafted with earth-based elements that promote healing and engage the senses of smell, sight, touch, sound, or taste. Queendom Qare is here to guide you along your journey to Divine Health through our signature line of products that promote *Divine SelfQare*.

Divine SelfQare Practitioners are women equipped to navigate a world of change fully in tune with their own minds, bodies, and spirits for optimal performance. You are now able to join the revolution to strive for Divine Health through *Divine SelfQare*. Now that you know this Divine Knowledge and have access to its sacred assets, you can create your very own at-home spa and take your health and wellness back into your own hands.

For more information and useful resources, visit Queendomqare.com today. Watch this online space for Wellness Coaching, guided and self-paced courses, and future Queendom Qare Practitioner Certifications licensed doulas, midwives, and medical professionals. There is more to come! For now, take the time to immerse yourself in *Divine SelfQare*. Take total control of your body, mind, and spiritual wellness. You have the mental and spiritual resources to do so, and you deserve it.

Epilogue

Divine Closure

My Dear Grandchildren,

I have loved you since before you were born.

I wrote this book with the hopes of you reading it one day. It was the driving force that kept me determined to complete this important work. At the time in which I began to pen down my thoughts, I was yet to be a grandmother. My faith in the Most High, along with my promising son, Zakur, had always fueled my hopes of one day becoming the grand matriarch of a thriving family full of healthy granddaughters and grandsons. My vision of you all extends from my divine imagination out to nineteen generations.

I have addressed these carefully curated words to my future grandchildren, whom it would be the greatest pleasure to hold in my arms one day. Among all that I do not know, I still feel confident that my future grandchildren will one day be proud to pass on the knowledge that I have sought to share with them through this book.

Although this book was written primarily as guidance for my future granddaughters, I hope it becomes a source of wisdom for my future grandsons as well. It would mean so much to me to have you, as my prayed for grandsons, read and impart this knowledge to your future wives, daughters, and perhaps any friends who may benefit from the wisdom it contains. There is nothing more than I would like than for this book to be a gift for all the generations to come.

Beloved grandchildren to prayerfully come, when I started putting my thoughts onto paper for this sacred book to come to life, I told you how Divine Health is everyone's birthright and *Divine SelfQare* is for any woman who embraces it and embody its principles, precepts and pillars as a foundation for health and freedom.

I pray that the journey you took, navigating through these chapters together with me, has blessed you. I pray that it has filled your mind with timeless knowledge that enables you to experience Divine Health and fulfill your Divine Purpose in life.

From the early concept of Sankofa to the voices of our honorable ancestors, my goal was to create a Divine Roadmap for you, realizing that a grandmother's wisdom and experiences have the potential to bring hope, inspiration, and make all the difference in the world whenever they are needed.

I pray this book feels like a warm, nourishing bowl of Divinity Soup and that it comforts you. I pray that whenever you need a reminder of how sacred you are to me; or whenever you feel the need to stimulate your mind or restore your soul, that you will once again sup from its pages and feel satisfied of spirit. I also pray that it serves as a constant reminder of the unlimited favor, grace, mercy, blessings, and divine protection that presides over each of you as the sacred children of the Most High. I pray that you persevere and know in your heart that truly, everything is going to be alright.

With Divine Love,
Grandmother Sheila D. Brown
January 23, 2022

Enlightened Queen,

Prayerfully, the information you have digested has inspired you to take action and get in control of your health and wellness. But, if you would like to learn more about implementing the Divine SelfQare Strategies that you just learned in this book; or, if you are interested in becoming a member of our Queendom Qare community of divinely-led healers, visit us at www.queendomqare.com to hear more about our upcoming certifications and courses.

Plus, we have a special BONUS for you.
Use this coupon: (TAKEOFF20) to get 20% off your first purchase at the www.queendomqare.com online wellness shop!

Feel free to share this great discount offer with your family and friends today!!

Love and Light,
Sheila Brown, JD

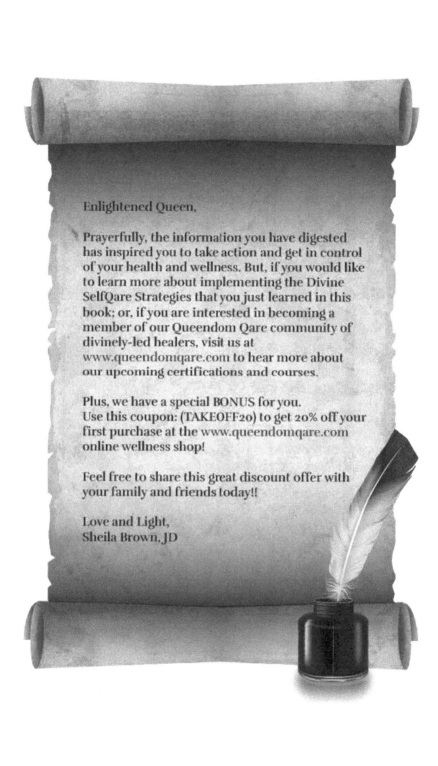

Glossary

A

1. **Addes** - *(Amharic.) Powdered lavender.*
2. **A.F.E.W.** - *An anagram for the four natural elements, Air, Fire, Earth, and Water.*
3. **Ancestors** - *A person or people, typically one more remote than a grandparent, from whom one is descended.*
4. **Alignment** - *The state or condition of being aligned with someone or something, a position of agreement or alliance.*

C

5. **Crown (also Qrown)** - *A term used in Divine SelfQare representing the head.*
6. **Centering** - *The idea of slowing down, finding calm in the chaos, and achieving necessary focus for oneself.*
7. **Candling (also Qandling)** - *The process of using the elements, air, fire and earth to cleanse the ear canal and experience a sense of spiritual and physical balance.*
8. **Cervix** - *The lower part of the uterus in the human female reproductive system.*
9. **Clitoris** - *The pleasure center of the vulva.*

D

10. **Dabo** - *(Amharic.) A term used for the female reproductive organ, also referred to as the vagina and/or womb.*
11. **Divine SelfQare** - *Reliance on the natural elements and divine intent to care for the body and mind.*
12. **Divine Health** - *The state of being in excellent physical condition, possessing a sound mind, and experiencing spiritual balance at any age.*
13. **Divine Intention** - *The good and pure plans of the heart and mind made before carrying out a task.*
14. **Divine Knowledge** - *The sacred knowledge given to us by the Most High.*
15. **Divine Closure** - *The concept of coming full circle.*

16. **Divine Listening** - *The ability to listen to the sacred first voice which is the voice of the Most High.*

17. **Divine Hearing** - *Being attuned to the spiritual ear through disciplined prayer, meditation and fasting.*

18. **Divine Purpose** – *Your sacred, spiritual purpose, as prescribed for you by the Most High.*

19. **Divine Speech** - *The concept of using your speech to attain your goals.*

20. **Duka** - *(Amharic.) A custom-built wooden stool with a large hole cut out in the middle of the seat.*

E

21. **Ear Qandles/Candles or Ear Qones/Cones** - *Queendom Qare custom organic candles used to cleanse the ear canal and instill a sense of physical and spiritual balance.*

22. **Emese** - *(Amharic.) A term used for the female reproductive organ, also referred to as the vagina.*

23. **Eye Mask or Eye Cover/Qover** - *An eye covering made with 100% pure cotton to facilitate thermal eye treatments.*

F

24. **Feminine Essence** - *A concept of a female who is in physical, mental and spiritual alignment with her own sense of divine beauty, creative ingenuity, and inner strength.*

25. **Foot Basin** - *A light and portable foot pool designed for soaking and relaxation.*

26. **Foot Soak** - *A blend of tantalizing salts and earthy herbs for the restorative healing of your feet.*

G

27. **Gabi** - *(Amharic.) A large heavy blanket made with 100% cotton.*

28. **Gojo** - *(Amharic.) A custom-built cottage for the process of smoking.*

29. **Gude gade** - *(Amharic.) A pear-shaped hole dug in the ground for the purpose of smoking.*

H

30. **Herbal Blends** - *A balanced combination of herbs for several benefits such as detoxification, cleansing, as well as therapeutic essences.*

31. **Hydrotherapy** - *a healing modality that uses water in various forms to create therapeutic health outcomes or enhance one's overall sense of wellness.*

J

32. **Jeweling** - *A therapeutic exercise to strengthen the pelvic floor using a pure rose quartz gem.*

K

33. **Kebi** - *(Amharic.) A thick butter made from cow milk.*

34. **Kemese** - *(Amharic.) A white pure cotton dress.*

35. **Kokabatis** - *(Amharic.) The ancient process of using smoky essence for womb wellness.*

36. **Kohl** - *An ancient eye cosmetic; similar to a black eye pencil*

L

37. **Labia Majora** - *A prominent pair of cutaneous skin folds that cover the labia minora, clitoris, vulva vestibule, urethra, and the vaginal opening.*

38. **Labia Minora** - *The inner lips; the inside of the outer lips.*

M

39. **Most High** - *The Divine Source; the Superior Being; Creator of all life.*

P

40. **Pedestal** - *A term used in Divine SelfQare representing the feet.*

41. **Plush Pillow** - *A lightweight, washable, luxurious pillow made with 100% cotton to facilitate all-natural wellness activities.*

Q

42. **Queendom Qare** - *An online Natural Wellness store housing essential product lines for head, womb, and feet care.*

43. **Qare** - *To care, replenish, and nurture your body and mind.*

44. **Qleanse** - *To clean, repair, and rejuvenate your body and mind.*

45. **Qrown Qare Steam Station** - *A portable steaming device designed for facial skin cleansing and nose/throat/upper respiratory detoxification.*

S

46. **Sankofa** - *A Ghanaian proverb meaning to 'go back and fetch it'; the Adinkra symbol that depicts a mythical bird, with a long neck outstretched backward to personify the proverb.*

47. **Steaming** - *The concept of using the steam released from hot water for relaxing and cleansing purposes.*

48. **Steam Gown** - *A white gown made with 100% cotton especially for steaming.*

49. **Smoking** - *The concept of using the smoke from burning special wood, plants, and herbs, for medicinal, renewal, healing, and relaxation purposes.*

T

50. **Throne Qare Steam Station** - *A portable steaming device especially designed for womb wellness.*

51. **Trans-physical** - *Of or relating to Trans-physics; Characterized or produced by the forces and operations of Trans-physics.*

52. **Trans-physics** - *Harnessing the power of Divine Intention to go beyond the physical properties or laws of matter, namely, air, fire, earth, and water; a spiritual type of physics; the spiritual form of physics rooted in nature's elements, activated through divine intentions.*

53. **Trans-physicist** - *One skilled in the spiritual form of physics as rooted in nature's elements and activated through divine intentions, a student of trans-physics.*

54. **Throne** - *a term used in Divine SelfQare representing the womb.*

55. **Throne Jewel** - *Certified Rose Quarts to help tone and strengthen your pelvic floor muscles.*

56. **Total Body Alignment** - *The idea of the body, mind, and spirit being in complete harmony as a result of Divine Self Qare.*

V

57. **Vulva** - *The vulva is the external part of the female genitalia. It protects a woman's sexual organs, urinary opening, vestibule, and vagina.*

W

58. **Wayra** - *(Amharic.) A kind of special wood.*

59. **Weybatis** - *(Amharic.) Another name for smoky essence.*

Y

60. **Yawre Abeba** - *(Amharic.) The biological menstruation process that a woman or girl goes through every month.*